Patient Safety and Healthcare Improvement
at a Glance

This title is also available as an e-book.
For more details, please see
www.wiley.com/buy/9781118361368
or scan this QR code:

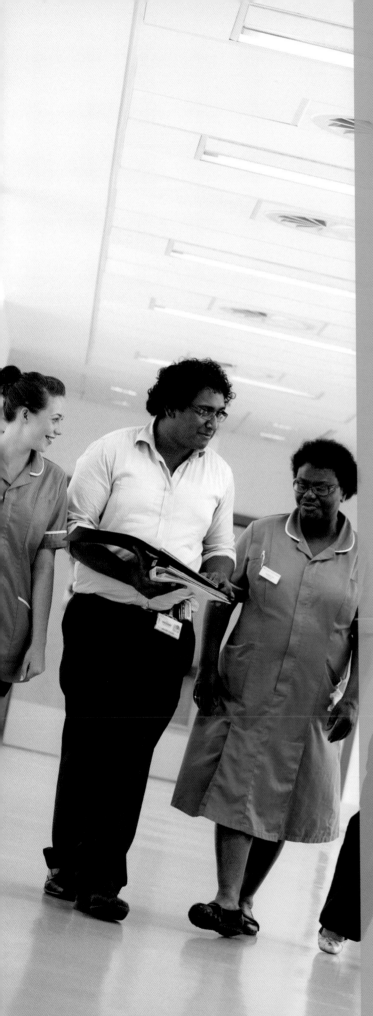

Patient Safety and Healthcare Improvement

at a Glance

Edited by

Sukhmeet S. Panesar

BSc (Hons.), MBBS, AICSM, MPH, MD
Honorary Fellow
Centre for Population Health Sciences
The University of Edinburgh
Edinburgh, UK

Andrew Carson-Stevens

BSc (Hons.), MB BCh, MPhil
Clinical Lecturer in Healthcare Improvement
Cochrane Institute of Primary Care and Public
Health
Cardiff University School of Medicine
Cardiff, UK

Sarah A. Salvilla

BSc (Hons.), MBBS, MSc
Honorary Fellow
Centre for Population Health Sciences
The University of Edinburgh
Edinburgh, UK

Aziz Sheikh

BSc, MBBS, MSc, MD, FRCGP, FRCP, FRCPE
Professor of Primary Care Research and
Development
Co-Director of Centre for Population Health
Sciences
The University of Edinburgh
Edinburgh, UK;
Visiting Professor of Medicine
Harvard Medical School
Harkness Fellow in Health Policy and Practice
Brigham and Women's Hospital
Harvard Medical School
Boston, MA, USA

WILEY Blackwell

This edition first published 2014 © 2014 by John Wiley & Sons Ltd.

Registered office: John Wiley & Sons, Ltd, The Atrium, Southern Gate, Chichester, West Sussex, PO19 8SQ, UK

Editorial offices: 9600 Garsington Road, Oxford, OX4 2DQ, UK
The Atrium, Southern Gate, Chichester, West Sussex, PO19 8SQ, UK
350 Main Street, Malden, MA 02148-5020, USA

For details of our global editorial offices, for customer services and for information about how to apply for permission to reuse the copyright material in this book please see our website at www.wiley.com/wiley-blackwell

Library of Congress Cataloging-in-Publication Data
Patient safety and healthcare improvement at a glance / edited by Sukhmeet S. Panesar, Andrew Carson-Stevens, Sarah A. Salvilla, Aziz Sheikh.
    p. ; cm.
 Includes bibliographical references and index.
 ISBN 978-1-118-36136-8 (pbk.)
 I. Panesar, Sukhmeet S., editor.   II. Carson-Stevens, Andrew, editor.   III. Salvilla, Sarah A., editor.   IV. Sheikh, Aziz, editor.
 [DNLM: 1. Patient Safety–standards.   2. Medical Errors–prevention & control.   3. Quality of Health Care–standards.   4. Safety Management. WX 185]
 R729.8
 610.28′9–dc23

                                        2014008376

A catalogue record for this book is available from the British Library.

Wiley also publishes its books in a variety of electronic formats. Some content that appears in print may not be available in electronic books.

Cover image: LTH NHS TRUST/SCIENCE PHOTO LIBRARY
Cover design by Meaden Creative

Set in Minion Pro 9.5/11.5 by Aptara
Printed and bound in Malaysia by Vivar Printing Sdn Bhd

1 2014

Contents

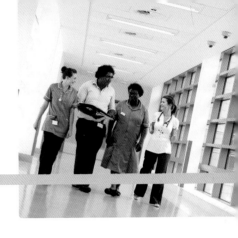

Part 4 **Quality improvement 67**

Contributors

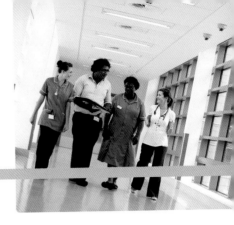

Elizabeth Allen
MPH
Postgraduate Student
Department of Public Health
Imperial College London
London, UK

Tony Avery
MBBS, PhD, FRCGP
Professor of Primary Health Care/Joint Head of Division
(Primary Care),
Faculty of Medicine and Health Sciences
The University of Nottingham
Nottingham, UK

Pierre Barker
MD
Senior Vice President
Institute for Healthcare Improvement
Clinical Professor Maternal and Child Health
Department of Public Health
University of North Carolina
Chapel Hill, NC, USA

David W. Bates
MD, MSc
Professor of Medicine
Harvard Medical School
Professor of Health Policy and Management
Harvard School of Public Health;
Chief of the Division of General Internal Medicine
Brigham and Women's Hospital;
Medical Director, Clinical and Quality Analysis
Partner's HealthCare System
Boston, MA, USA

Helen Bevan
MBA, DBA
Chief Transformation Officer
Horizons Group
NHS Improving Quality
Coventry, UK

Jay D. Bhatt
DO, MPH, MPA, FACP
Associate Physician Health System
Clinical Adjunct Lecturer
Department of Internal Medicine and Geriatrics
Northwestern University
Chicago, IL, USA

Maureen Bisognano
MS
President/CEO
Institute for Healthcare Improvement
Cambridge, MA, USA

Martin Bromiley
Airline Transport Pilot's Licence
Chair, Clinical Human Factors Group
North Marston, UK

Andrew Carson-Stevens
BSc (Hons.), MB BCh, MPhil
Clinical Lecturer in Healthcare Improvement
Cochrane Institute of Primary Care and Public Health
Cardiff University School of Medicine
Cardiff, UK

Ken Catchpole
BSc (Hons.), PhD
Director of Surgical Safety and Human Factors Research
Department of Surgery
Cedars-Sinai Medical Center
Los Angeles, CA, USA

Ashley Kay Childers
PhD, CPHQ
Research Assistant Professor
Department of Industrial Engineering
Clemson University
Clemson, SC, USA

Kevin Cleary
MBChB, FRCPsych
Medical Director
Director for Quality and Performance and Consultant
    Forensic Psychiatrist
East London NHS Foundation Trust
London, UK

Kathrin M. Cresswell
BSc, MSc, PhD
Chancellor's Fellow
The School of Health in Social Science
The University of Edinburgh
Edinburgh, UK

Mike Davidge
BSc, BCom
Director, NHS Elect
London, UK

Adrian Edwards
MBBS, MRCP, MRCGP, PhD
Institute Director and Professor of Primary Care
Cochrane Institute of Primary Care and Public Health
Cardiff University School of Medicine
Cardiff, UK

Lilly D. Engineer
MBBS-MD, DrPH, MHA
Associate Director, DrPH Programme in Health Care
    Management and Leadership
Department of Health Policy and Management
Johns Hopkins Bloomberg School of Public Health;
Assistant Professor
Department of Anesthesiology and Critical Care Medicine
Johns Hopkins School of Medicine
Baltimore, MD, USA

Gloria Esegbona
MBBS, BSc, MSc, MBA, MRCOG
Consultant Obstetrician and Gynaecologist & Lecturer
Department of Women's Health
Mzati Trust
Blantyre, Malawi

Donna Forsyth
MSCP, CMIOSH
Head of Patient Safety Investigation
Department of Patient Safety
NHS England
London, UK

Mark L. Graber
MD, FACP
Senior Fellow RTI International
Professor Emeritus SUNY Stony Brook School of Medicine
Founder and President Society to Improve Diagnosis in
    Medicine
St. James, NY, USA

Shabnam Hafiz
BS, MPH, MD
General Surgery Resident
Medstar Washington Hospital Center
Washington, DC, USA

Eric Hazen
MD
Instructor in Psychiatry
Harvard Medical School;
Director, Pediatric Psychiatry Consultation Service
Massachusetts General Hospital
Boston, MA, USA

Frances Healey
RN, PhD
Senior Head of Patient Safety Intelligence, Research and
    Evaluation
Patient Safety Domain
NHS England
Leeds, UK

Ross W. Hilliard
MD
Resident, General Internal Medicine
The Warren Alpert Medical School of Brown University
Providence, RI, USA

Aled Jones
PhD, BN (Hons.), RN (Adult), RMN
Senior Lecturer
School of Healthcare Sciences
Cardiff University
Cardiff, UK

Peter Klinger
MD
Instructor in Psychiatry
Harvard Medical School
Boston, MA, USA

Peter Lachman
MD, MMed, MPH, MBBCH, BA, FRCPH, FCP(SA)
Deputy Medical Director (Patient Safety)
Medical Director Great Ormond Street Hospital Foundation
    NHS Trust
London, UK

Tara Lamont
MSc
Scientific Advisor
NIHR Health Service Delivery and Research (HS&DR)
    Programme
University of Southampton
Southampton, UK

Susan Leavitt Gullo
MS, BSN, RN
Director
Institute for Healthcare Improvement
Cambridge, MA, USA

Carl Macrae
PhD
Senior Research Fellow
Centre for Patient Safety and Service Quality
Imperial College London
London, UK

Rajan Madhok
MBBS, MSc, FRCS, FFPH
Professor of Public Health
Department of Public Health
University of Salford
Salford, UK

Bhupinder Mann
BSc (Hons.), FRCS
Consultant Orthopaedic Surgeon
Department of Trauma and Orthopaedic Surgery
Stoke Mandeville Hospital
Aylesbury, UK

Ashley N. D. Meyer
PhD
Health Science Specialist (Cognitive Psychologist)
Veterans Affairs Health Services Research & Development
    Center for Innovations in Quality, Effectiveness and Safety
Michael E. DeBakey Veterans Affairs Medical Center
Houston, TX, USA

James Moses
MD, MPH
Medical Director of Quality Improvement
Department of Quality and Patient Safety
Boston University School of Medicine
Boston Medical Center
Boston, MA, USA

Mohammed Mustafa
BSc, MBChB, MRCGP, MSc
Clinical Lecturer in Primary Care and Public Health
Cochrane Institute of Primary Care and Public Health
Cardiff University School of Medicine
Cardiff, UK

David M. Neyens
PhD, MPH
Assistant Professor
Department of Industrial Engineering
Clemson University
Clemson, SC, USA

C. Jane Norman
BA, MBA, CQE
President
Profound Knowledge Products (PKP Inc.)
Austin, TX, USA

Clifford L. Norman
MA
Partner, Associates in Process Improvement (API)
Austin, TX, USA

Sukhmeet S. Panesar
BSc (Hons.), MBBS, AICSM, MPH, MD
Honorary Fellow
The Centre for Population Health Sciences
The University of Edinburgh
Edinburgh, UK

Gareth J. Parry
BSc, MSc, PhD
Senior Scientist
Institute for Healthcare Improvement
Cambridge, MA, USA

Velma L. Payne
PhD
Postdoctoral Fellow (Biomedical Informatics Specialist)
Veterans Affairs Health Services Research & Development
    Center for Innovations in Quality, Effectiveness and Safety
Michael E. DeBakey Veterans Affairs Medical Center
Houston, TX, USA

Susan Poulton
BM, FRCP
Consultant Geriatrician
Department of Medicine for Older People, Rehabilitation
    and Stroke
Portsmouth Hospitals NHS Trust
Portsmouth, UK

Valerie P. Pracilio
MPH, CPPS
Client Services Manager
Pascal Metrics
Washington, DC, USA

Peter Pronovost
MD, PhD, FCCM
Sr. Vice President for Patient Safety and Quality
Director of the Armstrong Institute for Patient Safety and
    Quality
Johns Hopkins Medicine;
Professor
Departments of Anesthesiology/Critical Care Medicine and
    Surgery
Johns Hopkins University School of Medicine;
Professor
Department of Health Policy & Management
Johns Hopkins Bloomberg School of Public Health;
Professor
Department of Nursing
Johns Hopkins University School of Nursing
Baltimore, MD, USA

Imran Qureshi
BSc (Hons.), AIEE, MBBS
BMJ Cinical Lead for Quality and Safety
Specialist Registrar in Medical Microbiology
Department of Microbiology
St George's Hospital NHS Trust
London, UK

Jane Reid
BSc, MSc, PGCEA
Professor, Bournemouth University
Bournemouth, UK

Kevin D. Rooney
MBChB, FRCA, FFICM
Professor of Care Improvement
Consultant in Anaesthesia and Intensive Care Medicine
Institute of Care and Practice Improvement
University of the West of Scotland and Royal Alexandra
    Hospital
Paisley, UK

Jane Runnacles
MBBS, BSc (Hons.), MRCPCH, MA
Consultant Paediatrician
Department of Paediatrics
Royal Free London NHS Foundation Trust
London, UK

Sarah A. Salvilla
BSc (Hons.), MBBS, AICSM, MSc
Honorary Fellow
The Centre for Population Health Sciences
The University of Edinburgh
Edinburgh, UK

Amar Shah
MBBS, MRCPsych, LLM, PGCMedEd, MBA
Associate Medical Director (Quality Improvement) &
    Consultant Forensic Psychiatrist
East London NHS Foundation Trust
London, UK

Kaveh G. Shojania
MD
Director & Associate Professor of Medicine
Centre for Patient Safety
University of Toronto
Toronto, ON, Canada

Debra de Silva
PhD
Professor and Head of Evaluation
The Evidence Centre
London, UK

Gurdev Singh
BSc Engg(Alig), MSc Eng, PhD(Birm.)
Emeritus Founding Director
Patient Safety Research Center
State University of New York
Buffalo, NY, USA

Hardeep Singh
MD, MPH
Chief, Health Policy, Quality and Informatics
Veterans Affairs Health Services Research & Development
    Center for Innovations in Quality, Effectiveness and
    Safety
Michael E. DeBakey Veterans Affairs Medical Center
Houston, TX, USA

Ranjit Singh
MA (Cantab.), MB, BChir, MBA
Vice Chair for Research
Department of Family Medicine
State University of New York
Buffalo, NY, USA

Sarah P. Slight
MPharm, PhD, PGDip
Senior Lecturer in Pharmacy Practice
School of Medicine, Pharmacy and Health
Durham University
Durham, UK

Lakshman Swamy
BA, MD, MBA
Boonshoft School of Medicine
Wright State University
Fairborn, OH, USA

Sundeep Thusu
MEng, MBBS, BDS
Clinical Research Fellow
Centre for International Child Oral Health
Kings College London
London, UK

Anthony Weiss
BS, MD, MSc
Assistant Professor of Psychiatry
Harvard Medical School
Boston, MA, USA

Preface

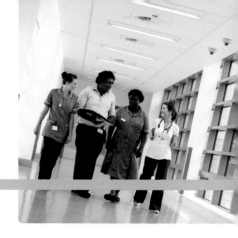

Healthcare improvement remains the bedrock of any adaptive, learning and high-quality healthcare system. The engagement of frontline clinical staff in advancing this agenda is central to ensuring improvements and safety in care delivery, thereby providing the best possible care for the patient. Since the 1990s, there have been concerted efforts to empower and equip healthcare professionals, carers, students and patients with the knowledge, skills and tools to execute and achieve safer, high-quality, patient-centred care. This book is an attempt to synthesise the key lessons learnt and distil these into practical recommendations.

Influential reports have raised awareness of healthcare quality and safety in the professional and public conscience. Seminal amongst these have been *To Err Is Human*, produced by the US Institute of Medicine (IOM), and An *Organisation with a Memory*, produced by the UK Government's Chief Medical Officer. These reports highlighted that error was routine during the delivery of healthcare and pointed to steps that should be taken to minimise their occurrence and the adverse consequences resulting from these system failures. The IOM advises six aims for quality – safety, effectiveness, efficiency, timeliness, patient-centredness and equity. A focus on patient safety has served as a 'Trojan horse' to create urgency for change and highlight the major underlying problems in healthcare, and in doing so it has galvanised the importance of seeking all the aims of quality. More recently, the Institute of Healthcare Improvement (IHI) launched *The Triple Aim* that challenges healthcare organisations to improve patient experience, improve population health and reduce the per capita cost of healthcare in order to optimise health system performance. Building on this approach, many of our contributors have used the lens of patient safety to highlight concerns about and approaches to enhancing the quality of care provision.

Our hope is that this text – which includes contributions from leading international scholars and clinicians in training – will meet the needs of healthcare students and professionals at all stages of their training: from students and junior doctors who have yet to be introduced to the disciplines of healthcare improvement and patient safety to those who want a quick refresher of core concepts and in areas that would be relevant for healthcare professionals in training. This reflects our core belief that all those serving at the 'coal face' of healthcare delivery have the capacity to be the barometers of the quality and safety of healthcare provision.

Finally, we are optimistic that all those who read this book will in some way – whether by initiating, leading or contributing to collective efforts – be inspired to move forward the agenda of safe, high-quality, patient-centred care. It is, after all, these enduring values that ensure we are fitting members of 'the noble profession' and that we, like every other generation before us, have fulfilled the charge of ensuring we take stock of preceding efforts, enrich them and then hand on these quintessential values.

Sukhmeet S. Panesar, Andrew Carson-Stevens,
Sarah A. Salvilla and Aziz Sheikh

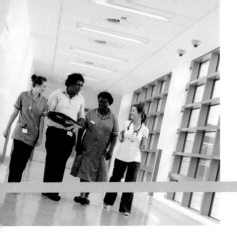

Acknowledgements

We wish to record our sincere gratitude to our contributors who have taken time away from their many other commitments to share their knowledge and insights. These wonderful colleagues have been a real pleasure to work with, and we wish them all the very best in their future endeavours. We owe particular thanks to colleagues at the Institute for Healthcare Improvement, Cambridge, USA* who contributed graciously to this book. Any omissions during the editing phase are ours.

We would also like to take this opportunity to thank our families for their support throughout the conception, gestation and delivery of this book. This work is therefore very much also a fruit of their labours, and we hope that they too will take pride in seeing the ideas contained in this book flourish.

*The Institute for Healthcare Improvement (IHI) (www.IHI.org) is an independent not-for-profit organization which hosts the IHI Open School (www.ihi.org/openschool). The School exists to advance quality improvement and patient safety competencies in the next generation of health professionals.

How to use your revision guide

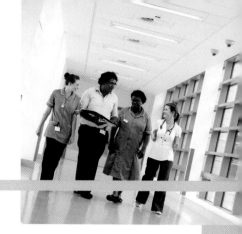

Features contained within your revision guide

Each topic is presented in a double-page spread with clear, easy-to-follow diagrams supported by succinct explanatory text.

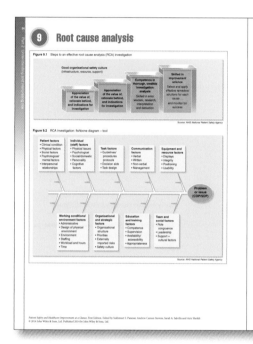

Your textbook is full of illustrations and tables.

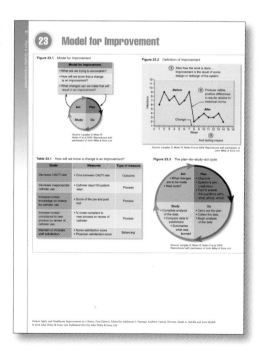

The anytime, anywhere textbook

Wiley E-Text

Your book is also available to purchase as a **Wiley E-Text: Powered by VitalSource** version – a digital, interactive version of this book which you own as soon as you download it.

our **Wiley E-Text** allows you to:

Search: Save time by finding terms and topics instantly in your book, your notes, even your whole library (once you've downloaded more textbooks)

Note and Highlight: Colour code, highlight and make digital notes right in the text so you can find them quickly and easily

Organise: Keep books, notes and class materials organised in folders inside the application

Share: Exchange notes and highlights with friends, classmates and study groups

Upgrade: Your textbook can be transferred when you need to change or upgrade computers

Link: Link directly from the page of your interactive textbook to all of the material contained on the companion website

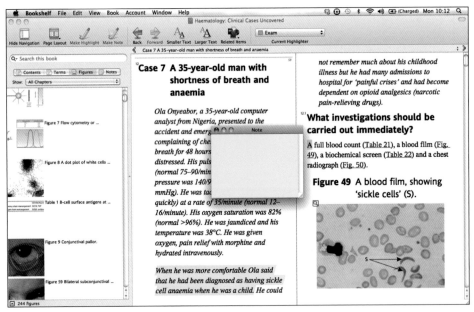

Wiley E-Text
Powered by VitalSource®

The **Wiley E-Text** version will also allow you to copy and paste any photograph or illustration into assignments, presentations and your own notes.

To access your Wiley E-Text:
- Visit **www.vitalsource.com/software/bookshelf/downloads** to download the Bookshelf application to your computer, laptop, tablet or mobile device.
- Open the Bookshelf application on your computer and register for an account.
- Follow the registration process.

CourseSmart

CourseSmart gives you instant access (via computer or mobile device) to this Wiley-Blackwell e-book and its extra electronic functionality, at 40% off the recommended retail print price. See all the benefits at: **www.coursesmart.com/students**

Instructors ... receive your own digital desk copies!
CourseSmart also offers instructors an immediate, efficient, and environmentally-friendly way to review this book for your course.

For more information visit **www.coursesmart.com/instructors.**

With CourseSmart, you can create lecture notes quickly with copy and paste, and share pages and notes with your students. Access your CourseSmart digital book from your computer or mobile device instantly for evaluation, class preparation, and as a teaching tool in the classroom.

Simply sign in at **http://instructors.coursesmart.com/bookshelf** to download your Bookshelf and get started. To request your desk copy, hit 'Request Online Copy' on your search results or book product page.

We hope you enjoy using your new book. Good luck with your studies!

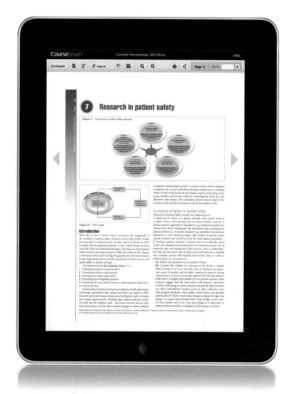

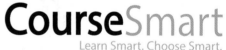

CourseSmart
Learn Smart. Choose Smart.

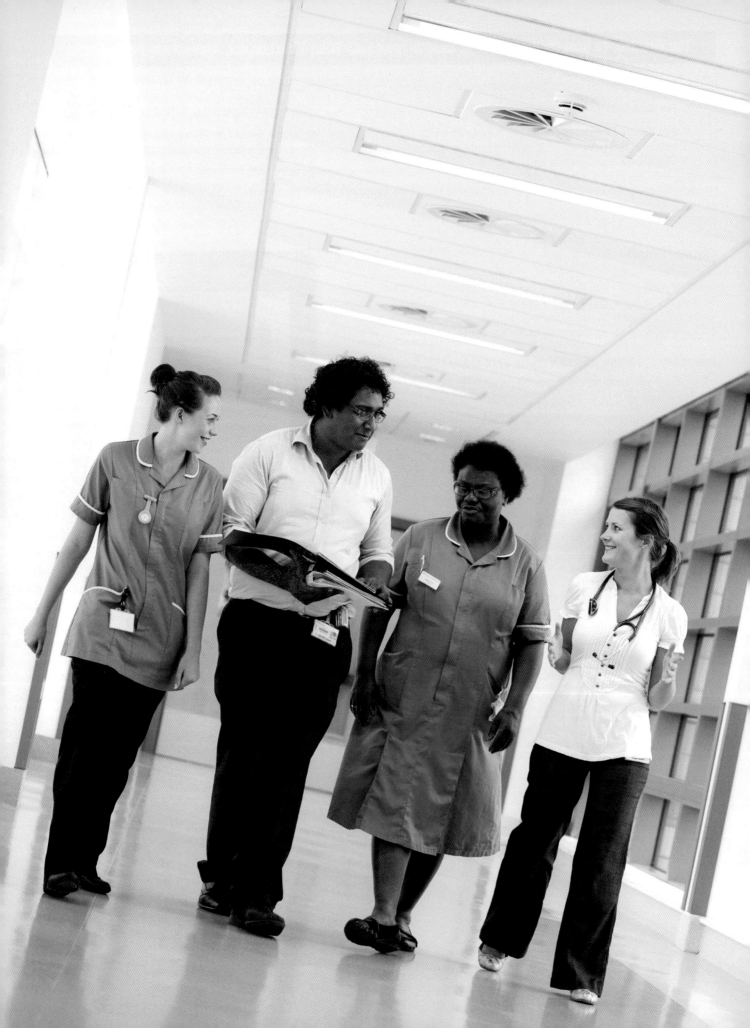

The essence of patient safety

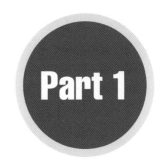

Part 1

Chapters

1 Basics of patient safety

Table 1.1 Patient safety terms

Patient safety term	Definition
Harm	Any physical or psychological injury or damage to the health of a person, either temporary or permanent Harm is usually classified as no harm, low harm, moderate harm, severe harm or death.
Near miss	Any patients safety incident that had the potential to cause harm but was prevented, resulting in 'no harm' (although this is a term of variable definition).
Adverse event (AE)	An event involving unintended harm to a patient that resulted from medical care. Traditionally, the term used for an adverse event was 'iatrogenesis'.
Preventable adverse event	An event involving patient harm as a result of wrong or inappropriate action ('error of commission') or failing to do the right thing ('error of omission').
Adverse drug event (ADE)	Any incident in which the use of a medication (including prescribed drugs, but also dietary supplements) results in harm to a patient. ADEs include adverse drug reactions (i.e. known side effects that occur even when the medication is used as intended), as well as events in which the drug has been used erroneously (prescribed at the wrong dose, administered in the wrong way etc.). ADEs that result from medication errors are often called 'preventable ADEs'.
Patient safety incident (PSI)	Any unintended or unexpected incident that could have harmed or did harm the patient. This includes 'near misses'. The term 'patient safety incident' is preferred to 'error', as the latter has a more negative connotation.
Critical incident*	A term first coined in the 1950s and made famous by a classic human factors study by Cooper of 'anaesthetic mishaps'. Cooper and colleagues brought the technique of critical incident analysis to a wide audience in healthcare, and followed the definition of the originator of the technique. They defined critical incidents as occurrences that are 'significant or pivotal, in either a desirable or an undesirable way'. Cooper and colleagues (and most others since) chose to focus on incidents that had potentially undesirable consequences. This concept is best understood in the context of the type of investigation that follows, which is very much in the style of root cause analysis. Thus, significant or pivotal means that there was significant potential for harm (or actual harm), but also that the event has the potential to reveal important hazards in the organisation. In many ways, it reflects an expression used in quality improvement circles: 'every defect is a treasure' . In other words, these incidents, whether near misses or disasters in which significant harm occurred, provide valuable opportunities to learn about individual and organisational factors that can be remedied to prevent similar incidents in the future.

*Source: *Cooper et al 1978. Reproduced with permission of Wolters Kluwer Health.*

Figure 1.1 Frequency of errors in medical care (adverse event rate)

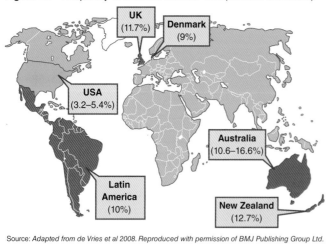

Source: *Adapted from de Vries et al 2008. Reproduced with permission of BMJ Publishing Group Ltd.*

Figure 1.2 The Swiss cheese model of how defences, barriers and safeguards may be penetrated by an accidentaly trajectory

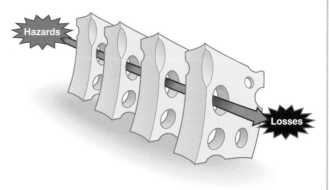

Source: *Reason J 2000. Reproduced with permission of BMJ Publishing Group Ltd .*

Patient Safety and Healthcare Improvement at a Glance, First Edition. Edited by Sukhmeet S. Panesar, Andrew Carson-Stevens, Sarah A. Salvilla and Aziz Sheikh.
© 2014 John Wiley & Sons, Ltd. Published 2014 by John Wiley & Sons, Ltd.

Introduction

As healthcare has become more effective, it has also become more complex and involves the use of new technologies, medicine and treatments. We are also now treating a greater proportion of older and sicker patients. These factors, coupled with decreased financial resources in most settings, can result in errors.

Two influential reports – *To Err Is Human* (1999) produced by the US Institute of Medicine and *An Organisation with a Memory* (2000) produced by the UK Government's Chief Medical Adviser – heralded the start of the global patient safety movement in the late 1990s. Both reports recognised that error was common during the delivery of healthcare: Figure 1.1 gives estimates of harm globally in hospitals. The figure of 1 in 10 patients being harmed is commonly quoted in the world of patient safety.

The reports drew attention to the poor performance of healthcare, as a sector, worldwide on safety compared to most other high-risk industries. Notably, aviation has shown remarkable and sustained improvements in levels of risk to air travel passengers over the last four decades. Both reports called for greater focus on, and commitment to, reducing risks in healthcare. In October 2004, the World Health Organization (WHO) launched a patient safety programme, in response to a World Health Assembly Resolution (2002) urging WHO and member states to pay the closest possible attention to the problem of patient safety. Its establishment underlined the importance of patient safety as a global healthcare issue. In other countries, specific bodies dealing with patient safety were set up: the National Patient Safety Agency (NPSA), which is now part of NHS England; the Agency for Healthcare Research and Quality (AHRQ) in the United States; the Canadian Patient Safety Institute (CPSI); and the Australian Commission on Safety and Quality in Health.

Despite these notable efforts, the current state of patient safety worldwide is still a source of deep concern. As data on the scale and nature of errors and adverse events have been more widely gathered, it has become apparent that unsafe actions are a feature of virtually every aspect of healthcare. Furthermore, there is a paucity of research on the frequency of errors and their associated burden of harm in areas such as primary care and mental health. Reports of the deaths of patients regularly feature in media reports in many countries and undermine public confidence in health services. Moreover, many events recur, with efforts to prevent them ineffective. These could be in part due to a punitive culture of individual blame and system failures. Initial, widely quoted estimates of the number of deaths due to medical error may have been exaggerated. For instance, a study by Hogan *et al.* (2012) of 1000 deaths at 10 representative UK NHS trusts found that only 5% were judged preventable, with 'preventable' being defined as having a greater than 50% probability that better care would have prevented death.

There is also growing concern of late amongst patient safety experts that despite all the efforts made to date, the patient safety momentum might stall as we have been at it for almost a decade and countless initiatives have been thrown at clinicians who may be overwhelmed.

Definitions

'Patient safety' can be defined as reducing the risk of unnecessary harm associated with healthcare to an acceptable minimum. An 'acceptable minimum' refers to current knowledge, resources available and the context in which care was delivered, weighed against the risk of non-treatment or other treatment. Simply put, it is the prevention of errors and adverse effects to patients associated with healthcare. Further key definitions are given in Table 1.1.

Concepts

The large-scale technological disasters on oil rigs, nuclear power plants and aviation in the 1980s led to more of a *systems-thinking* approach to developing safer workplaces and safer cultures. The same approach applies to healthcare; it is rare that a doctor or nurse is to blame for an error, but the environment and systems they work in play a strong part. James Reason, an eminent psychologist, developed the 'Swiss cheese' model (see Figure 1.2) to explain the steps and multiple factors associated with adverse events. Key points to note in this model are:

• *Defences, barriers and safeguards* exist to protect patients from hazards, such as alarms on syringe drivers or anaesthetists reminding surgeons to ensure that an adequate pre-operative work-up of the patient has taken place. These defences can be breached, like the holes in slices of Swiss cheese. However, unlike in the cheese, these holes are continually opening, shutting and shifting their location. The presence of holes in any one 'slice' does not normally cause a bad outcome. Usually, this only happens when the holes in many layers momentarily line up to permit a trajectory of accident opportunity – bringing hazards into damaging contact with patients. The holes occur due to a combination of *active failures* and *latent conditions*

• *Active failures* are the unsafe acts committed by people who are in direct contact with the patient or system. They take a variety of forms: slips, lapses, fumbles, mistakes and procedural violations

• *Latent conditions* arise from decisions made by designers, builders, procedure writers and top-level management. They can translate into error-provoking conditions within the local workplace (e.g. understaffing requiring the use of locum doctors). They can also create long-lasting holes or weaknesses in the defences (e.g. the intensive care unit being in a different building from the operating theatre)

Another notable individual, Jens Rasmussen, suggested that errors occurred due to deficiencies in *skills* (e.g. asking a junior doctor to perform a laparotomy), observation of *rules* (e.g. not washing hands before performing a procedure) or *knowledge* (e.g. being unaware that gentamicin levels need to be checked).

Subsequent chapters will build on the concepts discussed here and equip the reader with the knowledge to identify and rectify potential threats to patient safety.

2 Understanding systems

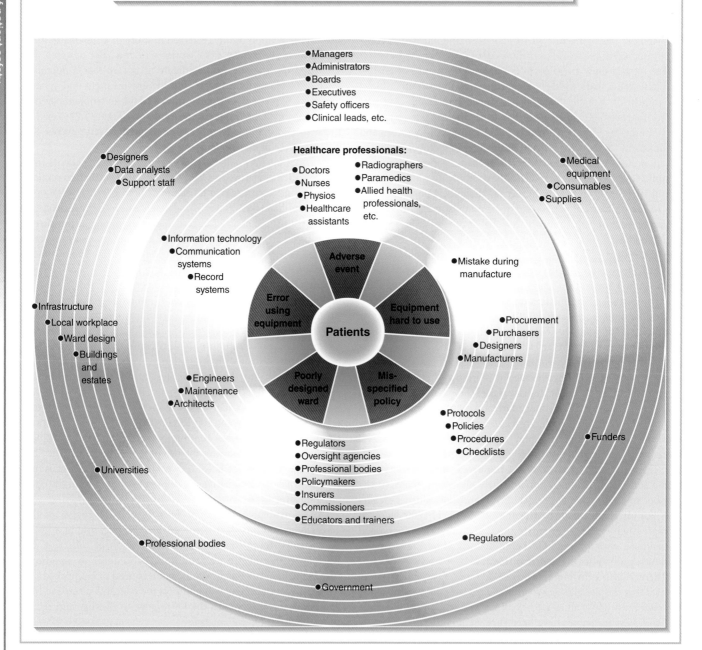

Figure 2.1 Healthcare as a complex socio-technical system and system accidents

The delivery of healthcare relies on a complex and wide array of people, activities and technologies

Each of these present opportunities for error, which impact on other parts of the system

Major accidents result from a combination of minor errors spread around these organisational systems

- Managers
- Administrators
- Boards
- Executives
- Safety officers
- Clinical leads, etc.

Healthcare professionals:
- Doctors
- Nurses
- Physios
- Healthcare assistants
- Radiographers
- Paramedics
- Allied health professionals, etc.

- Designers
- Data analysts
- Support staff

- Medical equipment
- Consumables
- Supplies

- Information technology
- Communication systems
- Record systems

- Mistake during manufacture

- Infrastructure
- Local workplace
- Ward design
- Buildings and estates

- Procurement
- Purchasers
- Designers
- Manufacturers

- Engineers
- Maintenance
- Architects

Adverse event

Error using equipment

Patients

Equipment hard to use

Poorly designed ward

Mis-specified policy

- Protocols
- Policies
- Procedures
- Checklists

- Universities

- Regulators
- Oversight agencies
- Professional bodies
- Policymakers
- Insurers
- Commissioners
- Educators and trainers

- Funders

- Professional bodies

- Regulators

- Government

Introduction

Modern healthcare organisations are enormously complex (see Figure 2.1). Even the most routine tasks of healthcare now depend on complex systems that connect a multitude of people, activities and technologies. For example, a typical patient in an intensive care unit requires 178 separate actions to be performed for them each day by a range of people, and a patient in their last year of life will typically be treated by at least 10 specialist doctors. The work of any individual healthcare professional is equally dependent on a wide range of other factors. These factors include everything from effective communication with colleagues to the staffing levels and resources within an organisation; and from the quality of equipment available locally to the design of wards and information technology (IT) systems. All of these factors and many

Patient Safety and Healthcare Improvement at a Glance, First Edition. Edited by Sukhmeet S. Panesar, Andrew Carson-Stevens, Sarah A. Salvilla and Aziz Sheikh
© 2014 John Wiley & Sons, Ltd. Published 2014 by John Wiley & Sons, Ltd.

more contribute to the safety of patients in any given situation. To manage and improve patient safety, it is essential to understand the nature of the complex systems that deliver healthcare, along with the ways that these systems shape – and are shaped by – the work of individuals. Safety improvement efforts need to be targeted at improving these systems. As human factors expert James Reason has put it: 'We cannot change the human condition, but we can change the conditions under which humans work'.

From individuals to systems

There has been a dramatic shift over the past two decades in how patient safety and error are understood in healthcare. Traditionally, if things went wrong, any investigation and remedial action would focus on the actions of individuals: typically whoever was closest to the adverse event at the time, such as the surgeon who operated on the wrong site or the nurse who miscalculated the drug dose. This view has now been replaced by a focus on the safety and reliability of the broader systems within which individuals work. 'Systems thinking' has long been established in other safety-critical industries such as aviation. In these industries, decades of detailed investigations have revealed that major accidents are the result of a combination of minor mishaps, inadequacies and errors that occur throughout organisational systems. The actions of the individuals who happen to be 'closest' to the adverse event are often merely the last link in a very long chain of events. This systems thinking underpins the entire field of patient safety, and was largely popularised in healthcare through two groundbreaking reports: *To Err Is Human* and *An Organisation with a Memory*.

Healthcare as a complex socio-technical system

Healthcare is a complex socio-technical system, in which even apparently simple tasks can depend on a wide range of social (e.g. psychological, team and managerial) and technical (e.g. equipment, IT and infrastructure) factors. For example, prescribing a medication depends on things such as IT systems that allow access to patient records, communication systems that allow effective transfer of information between health professionals, purchasing systems that ensure the pharmacy is properly stocked, education systems that ensure health professionals are appropriately trained and regulatory systems that monitor the safety and effectiveness of medicines. One defining feature of complex socio-technical systems is that there are many components and subsystems that must interact with each other to achieve a certain outcome. The effective interaction of each of the systems outlined here is essential to the safe prescribing of medications, and each is also a complex system in itself that requires careful management and design. Another defining feature of complex systems is that many of these components and subsystems are hidden from people working elsewhere in the system. The doctor who writes a prescription is unlikely to know much about the purchasing processes in the pharmacy, and yet all of these systems must function effectively together to provide safe care.

System reliability

Managing the reliability of systems – the ability of a system to routinely perform its function without failure – is a key factor in improving patient safety. Measures of reliability suggest that many systems in healthcare organisations operate at around 80% reliability. This is an extraordinarily low level. For comparison, if a car was 80% reliable, it would only work 4 days out of 5. Large commercial jets attain on-time reliability rates of around 99.5%. Low levels of system reliability in healthcare include:
• Systems that provide patient information for clinical decision making in surgical outpatient clinics operate at around 85% reliability
• Within prescribing systems for hospital inpatients, around one in seven prescriptions contain an error. One in five errors would have had serious consequences if not corrected
• Processes for ordering surgical theatre equipment operate at around 80% reliability. Half of these failures result in equipment being entirely unavailable

Much work needs to be done to make healthcare systems as reliable as those in other industries. This work is advancing rapidly, but it remains at an early stage. The Institute for Healthcare Improvement (IHI) uses a three-step model for applying principles of reliability to healthcare systems:
• Prevent failure
• Identify and mitigate against failure
• Redesign the process based on the critical failures identified

Organisational accidents

A particular challenge of complex systems is that they can suffer complex and serious breakdowns – 'organisational' or 'system accidents'. Minor errors and mishaps in one area of a system are not confined to that area, but can impact activities in other areas, often in unexpected and dramatic ways. Small mistakes can be amplified and have disproportionate effects elsewhere in the system. For example, a simple decision about adding a cleaning agent to a hospital's water system can have severe knock-on effects. In 2008, in the United Kingdom, one haemodialysis patient died and four others required blood transfusion after a cleaning agent was added to the hospital's main water supply. It had not been fully realised or properly communicated that the renal unit's water filters could not remove that particular chemical, which passed straight through into the patients' bloodstream.

Healthcare organisations increasingly rely on a variety of safety defences and controls to assure system safety. These defences aim to prevent errors cascading and aggregating throughout a system in ways that might cause a major system accident. However, these defences themselves can add complexity to the system, which in turn can introduce new risks. The water treatment process described here was itself being undertaken to address the safety risks of water-borne infection within the hospital. Safety defences themselves can sometimes introduce new risks, and safety improvements must be carefully designed and assessed from a system perspective to reduce this possibility. Healthcare depends on a complex, socio-technical system that can be challenging to fully analyse and understand. Improving patient safety requires a deep understanding of the many system interactions and system factors that produce both good and bad outcomes for patients. Every point of potential failure and error is also an opportunity for safety improvement and system redesign.

3 Quality and safety

Figure 3.1 Systemic constructs of quality and safety

(a)

QUALITY GUARANTEE

Timeliness   Effectiveness   Safety

Equity   Efficiency   Caring

Continuity of care   Patent centredness

8 dimensions of quality

(b)

SAFETY

Safety is a fundamental system property

Without safety there can be no quality of care

A safe organisation is a cost-effective quality organisation

Systemic threats to safety

- Complexity of the process of care
- Variability from patient to patient
- Inconsistency in the standards of care
- Poor interfacing (e.g. transition between settings)
- Lack of error-preventing barriers
- Lack of initiative to handle the unforseen
- Use of inappropriate time constraints
- Use of hiearchical culture in te system
- Human fallibility – *to err is human*

Lack of awareness of and attention to the above may lead to adverse events

(c)

Protective roof of quality

Assurance function

Donabedian's house of quality triad: structure-process-outcome

Flying buttresses

1. Interdependency
2. Organisational dependency
3. Consensuality
4. Congruence
5. Credibility

6. Relevance
7. Ownership
8. Mutuality of interests
9. Facilitation
10. Coerciveness
11. Virtue – personal and public

Flying buttresses

Efficacy | Effectiveness | Efficiency | Optimality | Acceptability | Legitimacy | Equity

Donabedian's seven pillars and eleven buttresses of quality

Patient Safety and Healthcare Improvement at a Glance, First Edition. Edited by Sukhmeet S. Panesar, Andrew Carson-Stevens, Sarah A. Salvilla and Aziz Sheikh.
© 2014 John Wiley & Sons, Ltd. Published 2014 by John Wiley & Sons, Ltd.

Introduction

The history of safety and quality started with the 'first do no harm' call from Hippocrates and the call for hygiene from Florence Nightingale. Despite various policies and initiatives, the progress towards improvement in this field has been unsatisfactory and demonstrates a need for systems thinking.

What is quality healthcare?

The quality of any healthcare setting is its total *system* characteristic. It is about doing the right thing (or things), for the right patient, at the right time, with the best results and at affordable costs. Quality has eight dimensions (Figure 3.1.a). A quality, cost-effective organisation springs only from a safe organisation. Overuse, underuse, misuse and the practice of economy with truth (fraud) are common challenges on the journey to better quality.

What is safety?

This too is a fundamental system property (Figure 3.1.b). Without safety, there can be no quality of care. It is one of the world's most pressing healthcare challenges. 'Safety' can be defined as freedom from avoidable injuries. Its goal is to avoid, prevent and ameliorate adverse outcomes emanating from the care processes. James Reason's trajectory of errors is an excellent aid to safety improvement because it helps in understanding the causes of failures in the form of *situational* (e.g. a very unusual work load, or a power supply failure at a critical juncture), *latent* (e.g. deficiencies in design, operation, maintenance, organisation and management) and *active failures* (e.g. human fallibility) that can result in adverse events, in the absence of appropriate technical (e.g. the use of informatics and safe-dosage packaging) and administrative (e.g. standard protocols and non-hierarchical team culture) *barriers* to this trajectory.

Similarities and differences between quality and safety

A quality healthcare setting has dimensions of safety, effectiveness, timeliness, efficiency, equity, patient-centredness, caring and care continuity. These can be seen as being housed in a protective Donabedian 'house of quality triad', which encompasses '*structure*, *process* and *outcome*' (Figure 3.1c). A *safe* healthcare setting, whilst being an indispensable and vital dimension of *quality*, is designed to face *systemic* threats of complexity in the process of care, variability from patient to patient, inconsistency in the standards of care, poor interfacing (e.g. transition between settings), lack of error-preventing barriers, lack of initiative to handle the unforeseen, the use of inappropriate time constraints, hierarchical culture in the system and human fallibility. Awareness of these threats leads to the ability to design and manage systems with barriers to prevent errors reaching patients.

The Donabedian framework

The triad of *structure ↔ process ↔ outcome* is a very helpful classification scheme for quality evaluation (Figure 3.1c). *Structural* quality evaluates healthcare system capacities, how the system is configured, and its components and their inter-relationships. Organisational culture and stakeholder satisfaction are also important elements. *Process* quality assesses interactions between patients and clinicians, as well as how care is delivered. The best process measures should be based on evidence relating better processes to better outcomes (e.g. controlling blood pressure reduces strokes and heart disease). *Outcomes* quality assesses changes in the health status of the patients and patient satisfaction. The best outcomes measures are those that are tied to processes over which the healthcare system has influence (e.g. the survival rate of pancreatic cancer is not a reliable measure as there is a lack of meaningful treatments affecting survival). Donabedian offered 11 essential principles (buttresses) to support the design, operation and effectiveness of the quality-assuring 'dome', supported also by seven pillars of quality (Figure 3.1c).

More recently, the Institute for Healthcare Improvement uses the term 'triple aim' to foster improvement at a systems level in three areas: improving the individual experience of care, improving the health of populations and reducing the per capita costs of care for populations.

Approaches to improvement

Because healthcare organisations regularly face new challenges, they must be adaptive to improve continually. Quality improvement in any setting is a systematic, data-informed activity designed to bring about improvement in healthcare delivery. All improvement approaches must meet three basic needs: (i) the creation of a culture of safety (Chapter 10) and a high-reliability organisation, (ii) the acknowledgement and treatment of each setting as a unique microsystem and (iii) the facilitation of workflow, processes and task assessment and improvement. There are *retrospective* and *prospective* methods of assessment for management of improvement. Widely used *retrospective* methods include error reports (root cause analysis, or RCA) (Chapter 9), internal and external audits, quality and safety indicators (Chapter 8) and trigger tools. Each one of these reveals only the *tip* of the iceberg of the quality gap and different perspectives of the same reality. Trigger tools reveal a much bigger *tip*, but are cost and time intensive. Generalisations of the results from retrospective methods can lead to stakeholder dissatisfaction. These methods tend to be top-down and do not fully meet the needs expressed in this chapter. The *prospective* approach is based on the failure modes and effects analysis (FMEA), as against RCA used in *retrospective* methods. FMEA has been widely used in other high-risk industries and has been advocated by the Institute of Medicine as a means of analysing a system to identify its failure modes and possible consequences of failure (effects) and to prioritise areas for improvement.

Human factors

Figure 4.1 Systems Engineering Initiative for Patient Safety (SEIPS)

Organisation
• Throughput versus cost versus quality
• Safety culture analysis
• Resilience engineering
• Accident investigation

Environment
• Noise, light and heat
• Interruptions and distractions
• Workspace layout
• Geographical distribution

People
• Selection, training and assessment
• Teamwork and non-technical skills
• Decision making and situational awareness

Tasks
• Task design
• Error analysis
• Error prediction
• Direct observation

Technology
• Product design
• Human machine interface
• Procurment and integration
• Technology surprises and risks

Patient Safety and Healthcare Improvement at a Glance, First Edition. Edited by Sukhmeet S. Panesar, Andrew Carson-Stevens, Sarah A. Salvilla and Aziz Sheikh.
© 2014 John Wiley & Sons, Ltd. Published 2014 by John Wiley & Sons, Ltd.

Introduction

The study of 'clinical human factors' is defined as 'enhancing clinical performance through an understanding of the effects of teamwork, tasks, equipment, workspace, culture, organisation on human behaviour and abilities, and application of that knowledge in clinical settings'.

The study of human factors, or ergonomics, examines the relationship between people and systems in order to build the working world around what people do well, rather than around technology or processes. By placing humans at the centre of our system of work, we can set about providing the best environment that will allow our best clinicians to perform to the highest level of their ability, or our least able clinicians (and there will always be a 'least able') to deliver care effectively.

This way of thinking originated in the 1940s and 1950s, when it was realised that the design of the displays and controls in aircraft could influence a crash, and thus sometimes made a difference between life and death. This understanding has been applied successfully to most high-risk industries and many consumer products. Good human factors enhance our interactions with the world so naturally that they are sometimes invisible.

The 'Swiss cheese' model

Perhaps the best known theory in human factors is the 'Swiss cheese' model (Chapter 1) of accidents where predisposing 'latent' factors can pile up on each other in unique situations to cause accidents, injuries and deaths. It is not adequate to blame lone individuals for making errors that lead to such catastrophes. Rather, we need to understand the predisposing factors that were always there, lying dormant in our system and only becoming critical when all these 'holes in the cheese' lined up.

This view helps us to understand that:

- humans are not the 'cause' of accidents
- humans hold complex and deficient systems together
- humans *create* safety in complex systems
- accidents have their roots in organisations, not individuals
- complex, high-risk systems are inherently unsafe
- accidents signify problems deep in the system
- problems can be visible but may seem innocuous
- accidents happen when problems combine

Thus, putting the understanding of people at the centre of the system provides a new way of thinking about how healthcare in the future might be better configured and delivered. The Systems Engineering Initiative for Patient Safety (SEIPS) model developed by Carayon and colleagues illustrates the system parameters that can influence human performance, and ultimately patient outcomes (Figure 4.1). The SEIPS model involves people, tasks, technology, environment and organisation, as explained in this chapter.

People

People are at the centre of any system, and they must exist at some level in the system to:

- design, operate and maintain technology or processes
- perform the key decision-making tasks
- work in teams to support each other
- circumvent poor processes
- avoid potential errors
- trap errors as they happen
- mitigate the effects of those errors

People prevent catastrophic failures and provide the key resources in the system that no machine or process can do. A greater understanding of what people do within our systems can contribute to training, or indeed help us design systems for better human performance. For example, the effect of fatigue on a range of human abilities has been studied for many years. We also know that performance at a task can vary with workload, where being 'under-loaded' can be as detrimental to performance as being 'overloaded'.

Human decision making is also of particular interest in human factors. In contrast to views of the human as a linear analytical information processor, we know that human decisions are not always linear, analytical or logical. Decisions may be based on situational factors (what is happening now?), system-wide decisions (what should I be doing?) and the needs of individual patients.

If we wish to improve how people contribute to the performance of the system, we can improve our ability to select the right person for the job by improving our training regimes or enhancing our assessment systems.

Non-technical skills and situational awareness

The introduction of non-technical skills training and assessment for surgical skills development can help to overcome some of the teamwork and communication problems that can predispose to surgical errors. These are grouped into:

- Social skills
  - Leadership and management
  - Teamwork and co-operation
- Cognitive skills
  - Problem solving and decision making
  - Situational awareness

Situational awareness describes how we notice information in our environment, understand what it means within the context we are working in, and are able to project into the future about where we will be. This emphasises the ability of experts to be able to accurately predict what may happen to a patient (e.g. deterioration) so the response can be timely and appropriate.

Tasks

Tasks define what we need to achieve a goal. For example, to get cash from a hole-in-the-wall, we need to put our card into the machine, type our security code, take our card back and get our money. How experienced we are with this task and how clearly it is set out will influence our ability to perform it quickly and accurately. In some instances, changing the order of the tasks can make a difference. For example, if the cash is returned before the card, there is a much higher chance of forgetting the card, since we have completed the primary task (getting cash) before we have completely finished.

To understand tasks, we can:
• use hierarchical task analysis to describe tasks that users need to perform to achieve a goal
• use human reliability analysis techniques and failure modes and effects analysis (FMEA) to predict the likelihood and consequences of making an error
• perform a direct observation to see what people do
• examine the difference between what is supposed to happen, what people say happens and what really happens

Once risks and barriers to the completion of processes are understood, it is then possible to redesign tasks to make them faster, more efficient, safer or less error prone. It is also possible to provide methods to assist with tasks, such as:
• sign-posting key processes to make tasks easy to do
• checking to ensure that errors are captured
• using standard methods to perform tasks consistently
• using checklists to aid technical processes
• holding briefings and debriefings to aid team processes (Chapter 5)

Technology and tools

A tool might be something as simple as a checklist or a pencil and paper, but might also be a complex imaging system or a device such as a surgical robot. All such technologies can assist the people at the centre of the system in performing tasks that will help reach their goals. The appropriate application of technology and tools can make work faster, safer and more efficient. However, technology that is not designed with the end users in mind can be burdensome and have the potential not to reduce errors, but to relocate them. Indeed, technologies are frequently introduced to increase efficiency and safety, but have the opposite effect. Common surprises with new technologies are:
• it doesn't replace the need for humans
• it requires them to work in different ways
• it requires them to work longer, harder or faster
• new skills are required
• different errors are possible
• different people may be better at using the new technologies
• it can de-skill people at the old tasks
• there can be an over-reliance on the new technology

For example, the growth in laparoscopy requires additional skills aside from the traditional surgical techniques, which in turn means that different people may be suited to the task. Although outcomes and patient experiences are generally better, it has also increased the chances of major complications such as bile duct injuries and, since open laparotomies are less practiced, they are more challenging when needed.

How the human interacts with the technology – known as the human–machine interface – can have huge implications for the likelihood of errors. For example, using infusion pumps side-by-side, each with a different design, will automatically generate the potential that the wrong buttons will be pressed and the machine will be set up in the wrong way. Training in the use of technology is also of significant cost, and appropriate or common designs can reduce these costs and improve safety. Thus, buying equipment that is designed around human abilities can result in substantial benefits that will outweigh the initial purchase costs. This has been convincingly demonstrated in the defence industries.

Another challenge with technology is in integrating it with the existing work systems, in terms of both the new processes and the new tasks required to effectively use the equipment. Maintenance and upkeep of the technology are also key factors that may be overlooked. Recent evidence suggests that the employment of human factors considerations in reconfiguring equipment may yield significant performance and behavioural benefits.

Environment

The study of human factors is also concerned with the effect of the working environment on human performance, such as:
• Noise and lighting
• Temperature and ventilation
• Workspace and physical location

Noise can be disruptive to communication or thought patterns, and can even be damaging to the listener. However, music in some circumstances may enhance performance. Lighting is an important consideration for clinical work, not just in surgery, and excellent guidance is available for understanding the optimal lighting conditions for particular tasks. Temperature and ventilation considerations also impact human performance and infection rates.

The physical organisation of the workspace will also impact human performance. Items that are too high or too low, that do not have a place to be stored or that are in storage that is disorganised, inconsistent or poorly labelled will be more difficult to access, therefore reducing human ability. Rooms that are too small to house equipment, supplies, teams or other necessary requirements of the task will increase risks and frustration, and reduce performance. They may also increase infection risk.

The location where work is performed is also an important design consideration. Bedside handovers may involve the patient, but are prone to interruptions and may have privacy issues during confidential discussions. Individual rooms improve patient privacy but may require extra monitoring.

Organisation

The final component in the SEIPS model relates to the organisation, which must support all aspects of the work environment. Considerations include:
• safety culture
• the balance between throughput, cost and quality
• organisational leadership and management structure
• preventing organisational drift
• learning from safety incidents and achieving a fair culture

Culture is often described as 'how we do it around here'. The assessment of safety culture can be particularly important in understanding the general consensus within an organisation about how people within it understand risk. A variety of tools are available for assessing staff perceptions of the levels of risk and safety at different levels within a hospital.

Cost and quality management

A key feature of any organisation's safety culture is the trade-offs that are required between throughput, cost and quality. Staff delivering care are constantly required to decide on the right trade-offs to make, and the leadership in any organisation will help to set the priorities. For example, key performance targets and measures for finances and throughputs with unclear quality or safety goals will lead to increased throughput and reduced costs, but at the potential expense of safety and quality. Making clear all three expectations for staff is a clear aspect of managing these conflicting goals, and a realistic approach to setting those expectations is required.

An organisation that takes an active approach to monitoring and adjusting staff expectations in relation to these goals is more likely to be successful in managing these targets. An organisation that fails to recognise when safety is being traded for other aspects of system performance can be prone to 'organisational drift', where safety standards become more and more relaxed until a serious tragedy occurs. In contrast, resilient organisations demonstrate resistance to these breaches in safety.

Learning from incidents

A carotid endarterectomy was underway with a 65-year-old male under local anaesthetic. Everything had gone smoothly and nothing appeared to be unusual. The consultant anaesthetist left theatre briefly to use the telephone. While he was outside, the surgeon asked for the heparin to be given, and the anaesthetic registrar picked up the syringe from the workstation and gave the medication. A short time later, the consultant anaesthetist returned, and asked about the heparin. The registrar informed him that it had been given, at which the consultant expressed surprise, and pointed to the syringe that he had prepared with heparin before leaving theatre. Since the error was picked up before the cross-clamp was applied, and the injection had been of saline, no harm came to the patient.

Response to safety events will define the ability of an organisation to learn, improve and avoid safety failures and adverse events in the future. This might be in the form of a debriefing (for minor events), analysis of incident reports (for a range of minor and more serious events) or a root cause analysis (RCA) (for serious events and harm). An organisation that blames individuals, simply adds more checks or only requires staff to re-train in the wake of a serious incident is unlikely to have learned the appropriate lessons, increasing the chances of a repeat injury or other injuries. Looking deeper into a system can be painful, but an organisation that encourages a fair and open culture, where potential safety concerns are openly discussed and where a full systems analysis is conducted that avoids blame as far as possible (and includes consideration of all the components of the SEIPS model), stands a far better chance of improving safety and quality of care in the future.

Summary

The study and application of human factors allow a diverse range of ways in which to consider and optimise human performance, safety, quality and efficiency in any environment. Performance and safety are influenced by the:

- people at the centre of the system
- tasks they are required to perform
- technology and tools they have to work with
- environment in which they work
- organisation in which they work

These components also interact with each other – for example, technology changes tasks and may require different training. This makes the study of any one system extremely complex. On the other hand, it provides an excellent opportunity to understand and enhance the delivery of clinical care. The application of this knowledge is known as 'human factors'.

Teamwork and communication

Figure 5.1 Case study – Elaine Bromiley

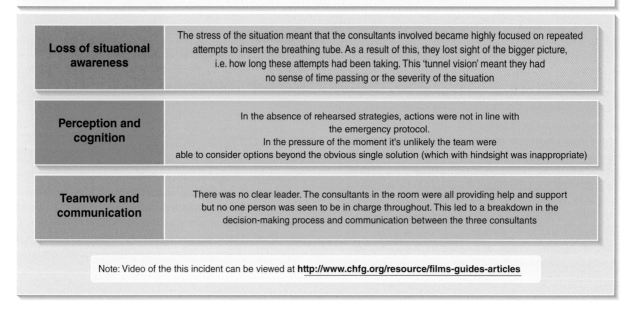

Elaine Bromiley was a fit and healthy young woman who was admitted to hospital for routine sinus surgery. During the anaesthetic she experienced breathing problems and the anaesthetist was unable to insert a device to secure her airway.

After 10 minutes, it was a situation of 'can't intubate, can't ventilate', a recognised anaesthetic emergency for which guidelines exist. For a further 15 minutes, three highly experienced consultants made numerous unsuccessful attempts to secure Elaine's airway and she suffered prolonged periods with dangerously low levels of oxygen in her bloodstream.

Early on, nurses had informed the team that they had brought emergency equipment to the room and booked a bed in intensive care, but neither were utilised. Thirty-five minutes after the start of the anaesthetic, it was decided that Elaine should be allowed to wake up naturally and she was transferred to the recovery unit. When she failed to wake up, she was then transferred to the intensive care unit.

Elaine never regained consciousness, and after 13 days the decision was made to withdraw the life support. Several lapses in human factors were noted:

Loss of situational awareness	The stress of the situation meant that the consultants involved became highly focused on repeated attempts to insert the breathing tube. As a result of this, they lost sight of the bigger picture, i.e. how long these attempts had been taking. This 'tunnel vision' meant they had no sense of time passing or the severity of the situation
Perception and cognition	In the absence of rehearsed strategies, actions were not in line with the emergency protocol. In the pressure of the moment it's unlikely the team were able to consider options beyond the obvious single solution (which with hindsight was inappropriate)
Teamwork and communication	There was no clear leader. The consultants in the room were all providing help and support but no one person was seen to be in charge throughout. This led to a breakdown in the decision-making process and communication between the three consultants

Note: Video of the this incident can be viewed at **http://www.chfg.org/resource/films-guides-articles**

Figure 5.2 SBAR in action

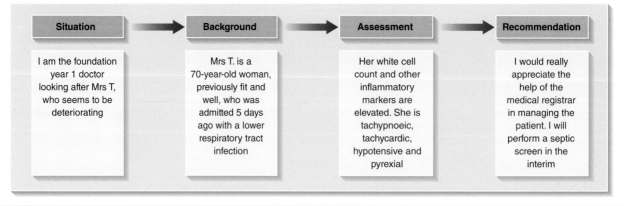

Situation	Background	Assessment	Recommendation
I am the foundation year 1 doctor looking after Mrs T, who seems to be deteriorating	Mrs T. is a 70-year-old woman, previously fit and well, who was admitted 5 days ago with a lower respiratory tract infection	Her white cell count and other inflammatory markers are elevated. She is tachypnoeic, tachycardic, hypotensive and pyrexial	I would really appreciate the help of the medical registrar in managing the patient. I will perform a septic screen in the interim

Introduction

A leading and recognised cause of medical failure is when teamwork and communication break down. As care becomes more and more complex, healthcare providers must work in large teams, often working across multiple sites or settings. In healthcare, a significant percentage of errors can be attributed to communication failures and ineffective teamwork. The Joint Commission has identified both elements as the primary root cause in more than 70% of sentinel (never) events from 1995 to 2003. Despite the critical roles that teamwork and communication play in the delivery of healthcare, professionals are not necessarily trained in these, and, as a consequence, a wide variation can occur in the quality of professionals' non-technical skills such as communication, situational awareness, decision making and teamwork. Effective communication and teamwork are essential for achieving high-reliability organisations and promoting a culture of openness and delivery of safer care.

Communication

Two approaches define communication: the 'information engineering' approach and the 'social construction' approach.

The information engineering approach defines communication as the 'linear transmission of messages through a conduit', that is, effective communication is the accurate transmission of information, resulting in the receiver understanding what is said. Noise (both audible and psychological) is the main barrier to effective communication in this model.

Social construction theory examines the way in which people work, their inter-relationships and behaviours in a team context and how this positively or adversely impacts the quality of team communication. This theory implies that communication is a social process. So much so, that efforts to improve the transfer of information are limited, unless the ways teams work, their dynamics and relationships are considered in parallel. Team communication is, therefore, not just about transmitting information but also about the social process of receiving that information.

Teamwork

The key features of a team are:
• It consists of two or more individuals
• Each individual has a specific role or task to perform and interacts and/or coordinates with other members to achieve a common goal or outcome
• A team makes decisions
• It embodies specialised knowledge and skills, often functioning with a high workload
• It exhibits interdependencies with regard to workflow, collective action and goals
• It is a part of a larger organisational system

There is a tendency in healthcare for teams to be organised hierarchically or geographically. Research highlights hierarchy, inhibits psychological safety adversely impacting the quality of teamwork and communication whilst teams organised across geography have to compensate barriers such as time differentials and distance. However organised, the priority is for teams to be co-ordinated and co-operative. Members of a team must engage in both task work and teamwork processes to achieve their common goal. Task work is the component of the individual member's performance that is independent of interaction with other members. Teamwork is the interdependent component of performance that is necessary to effectively co-ordinate the performance of multiple team members. Team performance is a multilevel process that develops as members engage in task work and teamwork.

The characteristics of an effective team include elements of:
• *Organisational structure* – clear purpose, appropriate culture, specified task, distinct roles, suitable leadership, relevant members and adequate resources
• Individual contribution – self-knowledge, trust, commitment and flexibility
• Team processes – co-ordination, communication, cohesion, decision making, conflict management, social relationships and performance feedback

The case study in Figure 5.1 shows how teamwork and communication can fail and result in patient death.

Tools to improve teamwork and communication

• *Briefings*: When comprehensively performed, these are crucial and determine how cohesive a team is when working on a task. They are initiated at the start of a task and set the tone for team interaction, ensuring that care providers have a shared mental model of what is going to happen during a process, identify any risk points and plan for contingencies. When done effectively, briefings can establish predictability, reduce interruptions, prevent delays and build better working relationships
• *Debriefings*: These are short exchanges that occur at the end of a task to identify what happened, what was learned and how improvements can be made for the next occasion
• *SBAR*: This acronym stands for situation, background, assessment and recommendation, and it provides a structured approach to conveying information to a colleague. Regular use of SBAR has been shown to reduce the number of patient safety incidents. An example of SBAR in action is shown in Figure 5.2

Conclusion

It is worth remembering that analysis of errors and the omissions contributing to patient harm, illustrate that the quality of clinical skills or discrete clinical interventions are rarely the root causes. Evidence suggests in fact, that the major causal factors of avoidable harm are due to the cumulative impacts of poor communication and sub-optimal teamwork.

6 Reporting and learning from errors

Figure 6.1 From reporting to learning

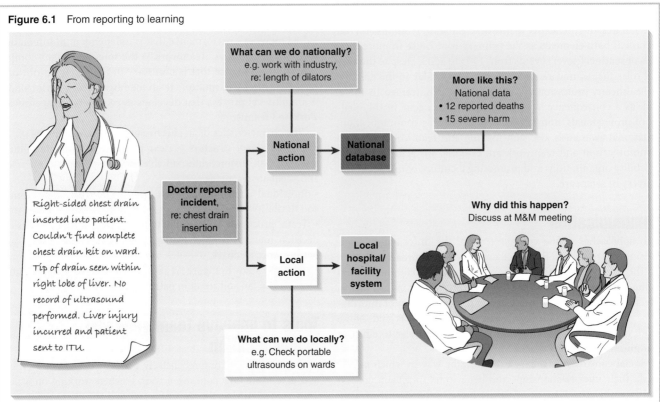

Introduction

Doctors and nurses are asked to report when things go wrong, so that others can learn from their experiences. Analysis of the event which harmed or could have harmed a patient can help to uncover important system weaknesses. Action can be taken at local and national levels to strengthen systems and prevent further errors. National reporting data also help to monitor risks over time and establish patterns of events (e.g. 'hotspots' following changes to delivery of home oxygen services) as well as common learning from rare events which may not be seen at every hospital. One Australian study showed that only 10% of all incidents that are reported nationally will be seen more than once every 2 months in an average 250-bed hospital. The remaining 90% of incidents would occur less often and cover 500 different kinds of events.

Reporting without learning serves no purpose. Reporting systems need to include a sense-making function, which looks for clues in the partial accounts from busy healthcare staff and brings incidents together with other sources of information and clinical experience to think about ways of making systems safer. At a local level, forums like mortality and morbidity (M&M) meetings in hospitals often focus on the single adverse event, or 'near-miss', to draw out common problems and unsafe practices. These are usually held monthly, and teams come together to discuss serious untoward events. At a national level, work can be done to standardise processes or 'design out' errors – for instance, changing the name of 'sound-alike' drugs (Figure 6.1).

How to report incidents

Each hospital and healthcare facility has a local reporting system, collecting paper or e-incident forms through a central risk management function. Since 2004, all NHS organisations in England and Wales have been connected to a national reporting system which automatically uploads locally reported incidents to a central database. Around 100,000 incidents a month are reported in this way, making it the most comprehensive national reporting system in the world.

Most healthcare systems now have incident-monitoring systems:
- Spain (ISMP-Spain)
- Denmark (Danish Society for Patient Safety)
- Sweden (National Board of Health and Welfare)
- Netherlands (managed by the Dutch Health Care Inspectorate)
- France (REEM, Preventing what is preventable in medicine)
- United States: state-wide systems (e.g. Pennsylvania State Reporting System), provider-based systems (e.g. Veterans Association) and theme-based systems (e.g. medication; Institute for Safe Medication Practice)

Some are voluntary systems, depending on professional codes of sharing learning. Other countries have reporting systems which are mandatory for all types of incidents (Denmark, Ireland, Czech Republic and some US states) or for deaths and cases of serious harm (Japan, Netherlands and Sweden). Although England and Wales have a voluntary system, organisations are required to report 'never events' – certain serious avoidable errors, such as wrong-site

Patient Safety and Healthcare Improvement at a Glance, First Edition. Edited by Sukhmeet S. Panesar, Andrew Carson-Stevens, Sarah A. Salvilla and Aziz Sheikh
© 2014 John Wiley & Sons, Ltd. Published 2014 by John Wiley & Sons, Ltd.

surgery. There has been little robust research comparing mandatory and voluntary systems and their impact on the rates, type and quality of reporting by clinical staff.

In addition to local and national systems, some specialties have bespoke reporting systems. For instance, a tailored anaesthetics e-form has been developed in England and Wales with particular prompts on common errors such as failed intubation and anaphylaxis. Reported incidents are analysed by anaesthetists to make sense of risks and identify areas for action.

As well as short incidents captured in real time by staff, more serious incidents may be subject to more detailed scrutiny. Avoidable deaths or serious near misses may be subject to local investigations, using techniques such as root cause analysis. This intense focus on a few critical incidents, taking evidence from many sources to identify system weaknesses, is more akin to reporting systems from high-risk industries, from oil rigs to chemical plants. Indeed, the first system to investigate error was developed in the 1940s to improve the safety and performance of military pilots. In healthcare, other kinds of reporting include local significant event auditing in general practice, where staff are encouraged to identify incidents from which others can learn.

Barriers to reporting

Research has identified a number of barriers to reporting – particularly from doctors, who report in smaller numbers than nurses. These include lack of familiarity with the reporting process, uncertainty as to what should be reported (e.g. certain categories of error such as omitted medicines) and scepticism that positive action will be taken by the organisation. There may also be cultural factors that inhibit reporting – fear of punitive action or discrimination. Qualitative research also confirms deeply held beliefs that may deter reporting by medical staff – that only bad doctors make mistakes.

What difference has it made?

Modern healthcare is complex and relies on multiple interactions between staff, and complicated processes and treatments. Reporting incidents where patients have been harmed or almost harmed ('near misses') is invaluable in pinpointing system vulnerabilities. Incidents reported locally might include equipment shortages on a crash call trolley or confusion from using different kinds of heparin. At a local level, actions might include an audit of resuscitation equipment and rationalising purchasing of heparins within the trust.

At a national level, steps can also be taken to make practice safer. This might mean standardising procedures (e.g. introducing a single crash call number of 2222 in all hospitals) or working with manufacturers to change packaging (e.g. more distinct forms of diamorphine to prevent wrong dose errors). In England and Wales, a national patient safety function has issued guidance on a range of issues, from chest drain insertion to over-sedation by midazolam.

Problems with reporting

There are limits to the value of reporting systems. Critics have pointed to low levels of reporting, with inherent bias due to under-reporting from key sectors, such as primary care which constitutes less than 5% of all reports (although nine in 10 healthcare contacts are in primary care). Studies comparing data from incident reporting with case note review showed that reporting was relatively weak at identifying some of the more serious incidents (although probably providing richer contextual information). This is confirmed by a US overview which estimated that only 5–20% of adverse events in different settings were reported.

There are also systematic biases due to who reports. Most reports come from nurses, and this is reflected in the type of incidents reported, most commonly patient falls. Many reports are incomplete, leading to data quality issues on coding of harm and sufficient description to act. Systems which are anonymous, rather than confidential, limit the ability of organisations to go back to reporters for more information. Despite concerns about underreporting, the large volume of incidents makes it difficult to identify the critical incidents which could be prevented.

Where do we go from here?

Research suggests that reporting systems are only effective with strong feedback loops and evidence of action following reported harm. In order to act on risks identified from reports, mechanisms are needed where clinical and other staff can interpret the story of the incident, combining this with other information on the clinical risk (from sources such as patient complaints or litigation data), and identify actions that will reduce risk. This can happen at a national level – for instance, action by professional bodies and manufacturers on spinal connectors following reported errors of intravenous medicines given by the wrong route. Action can also be taken locally, through reflection and multi-professional learning in forums such as mortality and morbidity meetings. Data on their own will not lead to safer practice. But data which are interpreted and understood, with an eye for strengthening systems rather than focusing on individual error, can transform practice. Each national safety initiative, from methotrexate prescribing to nasogastric tube replacement, started with a single report of patient harm from a busy clinician.

7 Research in patient safety

Figure 7.1 Framework for patient safety research

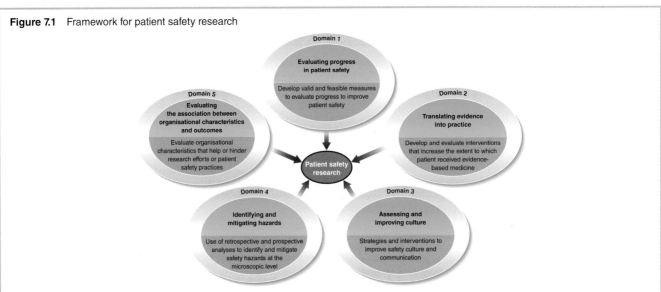

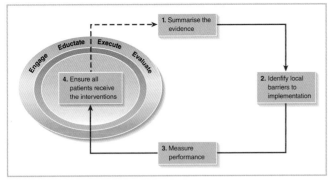

Figure 7.2 TRIP model

Introduction

After the *To Err Is Human* report uncovered the magnitude of the problem of patient safety incidents (more than 98,000 deaths per year due to medical errors), another report by RAND in 2003 revealed that hospitalised patients in the United States received only half of the recommended therapies. The framework for patient safety research and improvements (PSRI) described in this chapter evolved out of the need to bridge the gap between the interventions being implemented and scientific assessment of their success and applicability to similar settings.

The framework has **five domains** (Figure 7.1):

1 Evaluating progress in patient safety
2 Translating evidence into practice
3 Assessing and improving culture
4 Identifying and mitigating hazards
5 Evaluating the association between organisational characteristics and outcomes.

Besides these domains, tools such as simulation, health information technology, quantitative data analysis and others are useful in PSRI. Research and improvement must go hand in hand in order to initiate and sustain improvements. Hospitals must address both the technical work and the adaptive work – the former involves known solutions and science, and the latter requires changes in values, attitudes or beliefs to sustain improvement. A research study could be designed to address one or more of the above domains measuring or evaluating either or both of the technical and adaptive aspects, depending on the scope, timeline and access to data for conducting the study. In a collaborative team project, the centralised research team would do the technical work and the local team would do the adaptive work.

Evaluating progress in patient safety

Measures of patient safety involve two balancing acts:

1 *Balancing the desire of a global, although more biased, measure of safety versus a more focused, but less biased (robust), measure.* A global measure applicable to all patients (e.g. hospital mortality) has extreme bias due to inadequate risk adjustment and accounting for patient preferences. A specific measure (e.g. central line bloodstream infections) is very robust but targets only a subset of patients. Many specific measures are needed to cover the whole patient population.
2 *Finding a balance between a measure that is scientifically sound (valid and reliable) and feasible given the limited resources.* Use of relatively easy and inexpensive data sources, such as administrative data for measures such as deep venous thrombosis, is feasible but correlates poorly with medical chart review data. In order to address these, it is necessary to:

(a) Reduce the quantity but not quality of data.
(b) Consider the validity of a measure at two levels: a. Patient safety domain: If it is an outcome, does it represent an important aspect of quality, and do either variation in practice among organisations or interventions that improve the outcome demonstrate that it is largely preventable? If it is a process measure, does evidence suggest that the intervention will improve outcomes? b. What study design is used to measure the patient safety domain? Are there well-defined research protocol, data collection tools, well-designed databases, clear quality control plans, and detailed analytic plans? Cluster-randomised designs, a stepped wedge-trial design, or a quasi-experimental (time series) design can be used. As most studies tend to be a pre-post design, it is important to adjust for historical bias or changes in performance over time.

Patient Safety and Healthcare Improvement at a Glance, First Edition. Edited by Sukhmeet S. Panesar, Andrew Carson-Stevens, Sarah A. Salvilla and Aziz Sheikh
© 2014 John Wiley & Sons, Ltd. Published 2014 by John Wiley & Sons, Ltd.

Translating evidence into practice (TRIP)

The TRIP model (Figure 7.2) looks to improve the reliability of care by focusing on systems (how we organise our work) and engaging a multi-disciplinary team to assume ownership of the improvement project. It is based on evidence and performance measurement, and creates a collaborative culture that is essential for sustaining results.

Assessing and improving culture

The four important aspects of assessing and improving culture are:

1 *What is safety culture?* 'The way we do things around here' is a practical, easily understandable definition. Low-cost, quick, annual assessments of safety culture have led to a reliance on climate questionnaires, which measure a snapshot of the larger culture through different dimensions such as safety climate or teamwork climate. 'Safety culture' generally refers to an organisational culture, whereas 'safety climate' is more transient and refers to teams.

2 *How do you measure safety culture?* A Safety Attitudes Questionnaire is the most widely used instrument to evaluate staff members' attitudes towards patient safety. Unit/ward-level, department-level and institution-level assessment can be done around six scales: safety climate, perceptions of management, teamwork climate, job satisfaction, stress recognition and working conditions. Another widely used and tested instrument is the AHRQ Hospital Survey on Patient Safety Culture (HSOPS).

3 *How do you use safety culture results?* The two goals in assessing safety culture progress are to achieve or maintain a unit-level score of at least 60% agreement, and improve last year's climate score by 10 points or more (on a 100-point scale). Unit/ward-level results help hospitals recognise units that need resources or leadership support, and help health systems identify hospitals that are struggling versus those that are thriving.

Identifying and mitigating hazards

The following two methods are used to identify and analyse the healthcare system at the level of the unit/ward, department or hospital, to determine the source of potential or known risks to patient safety:

1 *Retrospective identification of hazards*: This involves in-depth analyses of sentinel events to identify the causes and contributing factors associated with an adverse event, then planning and implementing strategies to prevent the event from recurring. This may be formal (e.g. root cause analysis) or informal (e.g. case review by a quality improvement committee). Tools such as the 'Learning from Defects' tool help with in-depth analysis. Other tools include incident-reporting systems (e.g. the National Reporting and Learning System that collects reports of patient safety incidents); medication error-reporting systems such as MEdMARX, which collects data on medication errors in the United States; and intensive care unit safety reporting systems.

2 *Prospective identification of hazards*: This involves identifying hazards in the system before patient harm occurs. Unfortunately this is limited by institutional resources and capacity to accomplish the task. Failure mode and effects analysis (FMEA) is a tool used by the aeronautical industry but its validity, reliability and effectiveness have not been well documented (Chapter 27). Simulation is another tool which holds promise to improve patient safety; for example, simulation of resuscitation during cardiac arrest or mass-causality events helps identify hazards in the process of care.

Evaluating the association between organisational characteristics and outcomes

Organisational context must be taken into account in research, as social and structural characteristics strongly influence employee behaviour. For example:

- How to translate evidence into practice?
- What resources to dedicate towards improvement efforts?
- How to mistake-proof day-to-day operations?

Organisational variables that can affect patient outcomes are:

- Organisational design
- Organisational culture
- Policies, procedures and requirements
- Rewards and incentives
- Communication networks (formal and informal within and outside the organisation)
- Patient centredness
- Skills, knowledge and dedication of leaders

Knowledge about the association between the above characteristics and patient safety is important, but difficult to assess because valid measures of patient safety are difficult to obtain and organisational variables lack a standard definition. This could introduce misclassification and measurement bias (e.g. variation in nurse turnover definitions at the unit and hospital level).

Challenges for patient safety research

The following challenges need to be overcome in order to apply an effective research and improvement framework:

1 *Build capacity*: The only way to build momentum in the field of patient safety research is to provide trainees with formal coursework in research methods, mentorship and structured research experience. Advanced trainees are encouraged to get a master's or doctoral degree in their field of work. Due to the paucity of time, a start could be attending weeklong workshops to grasp the concepts. Evaluation skills can be obtained by prolonged coursework. In order to provide common guidelines for training in patient safety research, the World Health Organization has produced a guide to enable teaching across the globe in a standardised format.

2 *Create infrastructure*: A platform needs to be established for there to be an interchange between clinicians and methodologists. One way to do this is to hold regular multi-disciplinary meetings to bring the disciplines of clinical work and quantitative research together.

3 *Evaluate the cost–benefit ratio of improvement efforts*: Researchers need to be able to articulate the cost–benefit ratio of interventions, such as hiring new staff or purchasing new equipment, to enable the senior leadership and regulators to make informed decisions before mandating a safe practice.

Future direction

Key recommendations for future work in patient safety research are:

1 Develop valid measures to evaluate patient safety progress.

2 Develop methods to reliably translate evidence into practice.

3 Study the link between culture, behaviour and outcomes.

4 Evaluate teamwork and leadership behaviours.

5 Use simulations to:
  (a) evaluate teamwork and technical work
  (b) train staff
  (c) identify and mitigate hazards.

6 Coordinate national efforts to implement industry-wide changes.

7 Explore ways to effectively and efficiently use resources at all levels of a service (unit, ward, department and hospital).

8 Advance the science of measurement and reduction of diagnostic errors in medicine.

9 Develop patient safety measures for specific product lines (e.g. cardiac surgery) that should be mostly generalisable across settings.

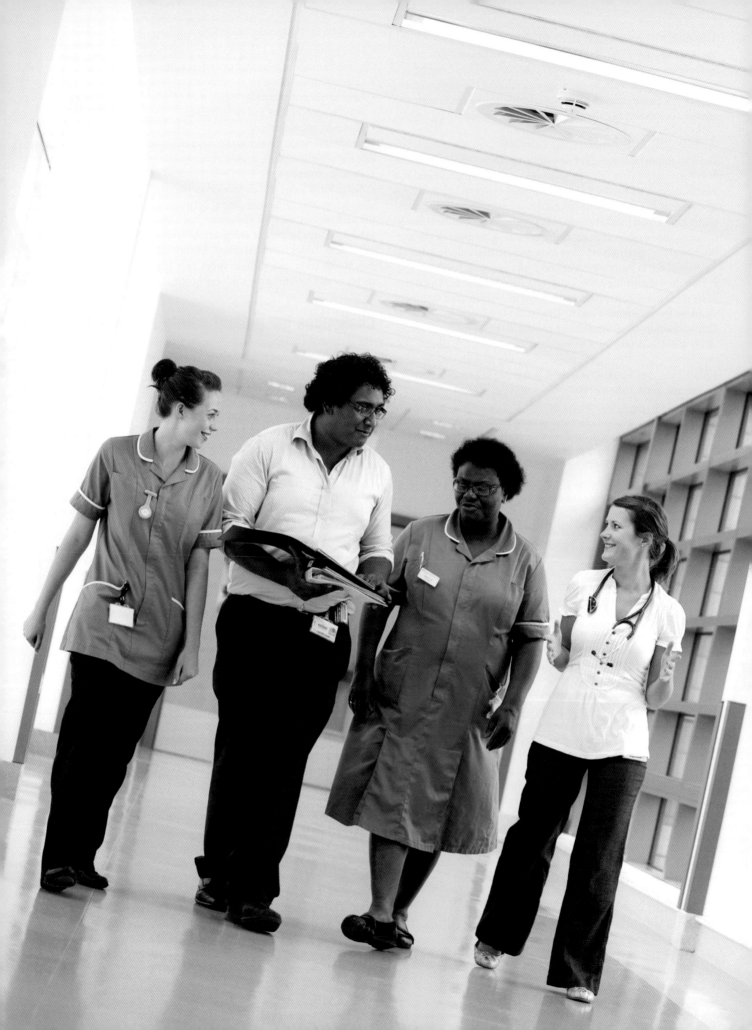

Understanding and interpreting risk

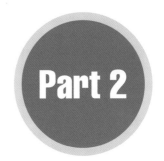

Part 2

Chapters

Risk-based patient safety metrics

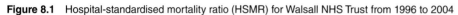

Figure 8.1 Hospital-standardised mortality ratio (HSMR) for Walsall NHS Trust from 1996 to 2004

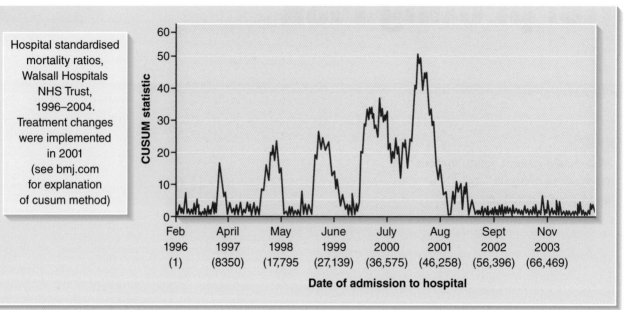

Source: *Jarman B, Bottle A, Aylin P & Browne M 2005. Reproduced with permission of BMJ Publishing Group Ltd.*

Note: Treatment changes were implemented in 2001. CUSUM, cumulative sum chart.

Patient Safety and Healthcare Improvement at a Glance, First Edition. Edited by Sukhmeet S. Panesar, Andrew Carson-Stevens, Sarah A. Salvilla and Aziz Sheikh
© 2014 John Wiley & Sons, Ltd. Published 2014 by John Wiley & Sons, Ltd.

Introduction

Patient safety metrics are measures of health service performance in the context of patient safety. They are the evidence base that guides quality improvement strategies to minimise harm and enhance patient experience. Patient safety programmes choose a metric this is based on available data, provides reliable and valid measures and supports desired objectives.

The two safety metrics most commonly used in healthcare aim to eliminate medical errors and prevent patient injuries. In industry, there is a third metric that focuses on proactively identifying and removing hazards to improve workplace safety. This last metric is not yet widely adopted in patient safety programmes, but may prove a useful systematic approach to design safer systems that support and enhance service delivery performance. The success of safety improvement initiatives is reliant upon these metric characteristics, as flawed or inappropriate frameworks can misguide strategies and have high opportunity costs.

Error-based patient safety metrics

Error-based metrics aim to detect and reduce medical errors, regardless of their impact on patient safety. The Institute of Medicine (IOM) defines error as the failure to complete a planned action as intended or the use of the wrong strategy to achieve a desired objective. This metric system attempts to capture both of types of error in the error rate measurement:

Error rate = Identified errors / total opportunities for error

The magnitude of this rate is compared to national or regional standards to determine the focus of improvement strategies.

Recent reports have highlighted the unacceptably high frequency of preventable adverse events and near misses arising from medical errors. Their significant impact on mortality, morbidity and healthcare costs makes this approach an important measure of patient safety and a useful guide for harm-preventing strategies.

Limitations

- *Imprecise error rate*: The accuracy and reliability of error rates are limited to the method of detection. Current methods are limited to voluntary reporting, chart review and direct observation. These techniques provide complementary results, but they are not independently valid, reliable means of error identification
- *Hindsight bias*: Retrospective error identification is susceptible to misinterpretation of events leading to poor outcomes, because the outcome is known. Inaccurate perceptions of causality can misguide improvement efforts
- *Reinforcement of blame*: A focus on individual rather than systemic failures does not address broader safety concerns that could lead to sustained quality improvements. Errors arise from latent and active failures; however, this metric only captures those from active failures, ignoring wider influences
- *Not always related to harm*: Many errors do not impact patient safety; thus, a focus on preventing errors may not lead to directly observable improved health outcomes
- *Negative connotation*: Health providers' fear of malpractice suits may cause a high rate of underreporting

Injury-based patient safety metrics

Injury-based metrics aim to eliminate preventable adverse events, including those that are not associated with any identifiable error. The injury-centred framework is based on the rate of injury that can be monitored over time:

Injury rate = Identified injuries / total opportunities for injury

Unlike error-based safety metrics, this approach allocates resources and sets safety priorities that will lead directly to observable improvements. However, this method is necessarily retrospective and reactive in nature, and is thus subject to similar limitations as error-based metrics and additional ethical constraints.

Limitations

- *Reactive rather than proactive*: Fails to proactively prevent harm by requiring that patients be injured before improvement measures are taken
- *Reinforcement of blame*
- *Poor discrimination of preventability*: Without a reliable tool to discern preventability, resources may be wasted attempting to prevent unavoidable injures
- *Imprecise injury rate*: Identification of injuries depends on routinely collected administrative data, which are often incomplete. It is also difficult to identify all opportunities for injury. Thus, this rate is susceptible to frequent random variation
- *Hindsight bias*: Retrospective approach makes it susceptible to oversimplified attribution of cause of patient injury
- *Negative connotation*

Hazard- or risk-based patient safety metrics

Hazard-based metrics aim to proactively identify, measure and remove hazards to create a safer work environment. This approach extends patient safety initiatives beyond individual-centred improvements to address the broader interacting healthcare system elements, including organisational structure, environment and technology. The premise of this method is that through designing a safer system, medical error reduction and injury prevention will follow. This metric system also has a more positive connotation than error and injury-based metrics and is likely to encourage greater physician involvement.

Limitations

- *Difficult to identify all hazards*: All potential risks to patient safety will never be eliminated
- *Limited use in the patient safety context to date*: There is little evidence of its success in the healthcare setting, although it is extensively used in industry
- *Impact on patient safety is not directly measurable*

Other applications of metrics

Death is the most tractable outcome of care – it is easily measured, is of undisputed importance to everyone and is common in hospital settings. This led to the creation of hospital-standardised mortality ratios (HSMRs). These are another useful tool to evaluate hospital performance by comparing risk-adjusted mortality rates with the national average. Hospitals monitor changing patterns in performance over time through a graphical presentation termed the 'cumulative sum chart', or CUSUM (Figure 8.1). This chart demonstrates how HSMR can be analysed at various time intervals to detect unacceptably high mortality rates and the success of subsequent improvement efforts. A hospital's HSMRs can then be compared to those of other hospitals, as shown in Figure 8.2.

Figure 8.2 Comparing efficiency and hospital-standardised mortality ratio HSMR for five hospitals

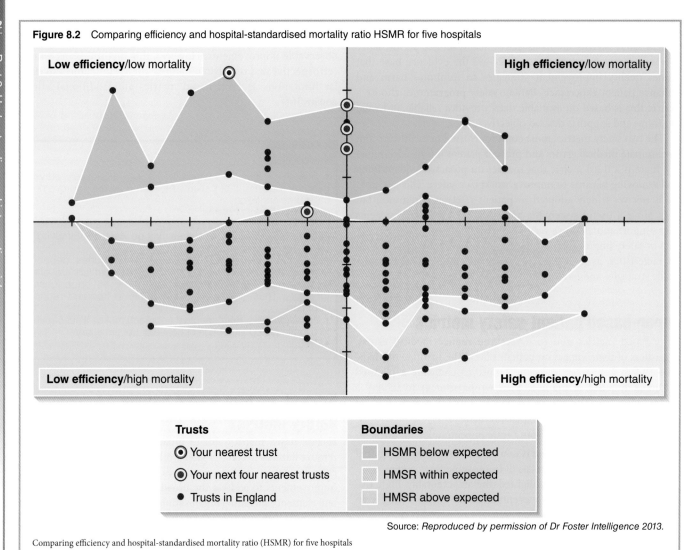

Comparing efficiency and hospital-standardised mortality ratio (HSMR) for five hospitals

Source: *Reproduced by permission of Dr Foster Intelligence 2013.*

A high death rate can be attributed to chance, regression to the mean, different procedures, inadequate case-mix adjustment, poor data quality or poor quality of care. All other reasons must be investigated before poor performance is considered the cause of the alarm. The advantage of using health outcomes to measure performance is that it is objective, readily available and routinely collected, and matters most to patients. However, this measure is also easily affected by confounding factors, includes unavoidable mortality, and is difficult to adjust for case-mix factors.

Quality indicators

Quality indicators are screening tools used to identify poor quality of care and patient safety concerns. These measures are based on routinely collected hospital administrative data that contain information on diagnoses, procedures, patient characteristics and discharge status. Although the data capture a limited picture of service quality, they provide a common denominator on which to compare hospital performance and guide quality improvement efforts.

Comparative performance assessments based on risk-adjusted quality indicators highlight unacceptable variation in health outcomes between regions, communities and providers. While quality indicators do not provide definitive measures of healthcare quality, they are starting points for further investigation and guide pay-for-performance incentives.

Types of indicators

1 *Patient Safety Quality Indicators (PSIs)*: These indicators screen for preventable adverse events and complications arising from medical interventions. PSIs can be based on a single hospital episode (provider-level indicators) or cases from separate hospital episodes (area-level indicators). However, it is difficult to distinguish preventable from unpreventable adverse events.
2 *Prevention Quality Indicators (PQIs)*: These assess the quality of health services in local communities (outpatient care) using inpatient hospital data. PQIs focus on ambulatory care sensitive conditions for which good outpatient care can prevent the need for hospitalisation. However, inpatient data do not consider patient preferences for inpatient and outpatient care, or socio-economic influences. There is also little evidence to suggest that effective outpatient treatments reduce hospital admissions.

Limitations of administrative data

- Fails to capture all complications of interest
- Prone to incomplete reporting
- Over-emphasises surgical procedures
- Hard to distinguish medical complications from comorbidities
- Collected for billing purposes, not for research
- Coding differences across hospitals
- Ambiguous timing of condition onset: codes fail to distinguish if it occurred before or during hospital stay
- Limited clinical characterisation: codes tend to group highly heterogeneous clinical conditions into a single code
- Limited case-mix factors

---

3 *Inpatient Quality Indicators (IQIs)*: These assess inpatient hospital care using in-hospital mortality rates; utilisation measures of procedures in question for overuse, underuse and misuse; and volume measures of procedures for which evidence suggests a link between the number of procedures performed and health outcomes.

Never events

'Never events' are preventable, serious and unambiguously defined adverse incidents that should not occur if appropriate national safety measures and guidelines are in place. They refer to alarming medical errors such as wrong-site surgery, retained instrument post operation and wrong route of administration of chemotherapy. Never events are warning signs indicating inadequate and ineffective patient safety systems that require further investigation. They are an attempt to chase zero avoidable harm in healthcare. Monitoring never events within the contract between commissioners and providers forms part of the wider safety and quality agenda in the English NHS and also in other countries internationally, such as the United States. Increasing pressure is being put on healthcare organisations to eliminate never events. In fact, the US Centre for Medicare and Medicaid Services (CMS) announced in August 2007 that Medicare would no longer pay for additional costs associated with many preventable errors, including those considered never events.

In the United States, never events are publicly reported, with the goal of increasing accountability and improving the quality of care. Since the National Quality Forum (NQF) disseminated its original never events list in 2002, 11 states have mandated reporting of these incidents whenever they occur, and an additional 16 states mandate reporting of serious adverse events (including many of the NQF never events). Healthcare facilities are accountable for correcting systematic problems that contributed to the event, with some states (such as Minnesota) mandating performance of a root cause analysis and reporting its results. Similar initiatives have been seen in the United Kingdom. In January 2012, the Department of Health published its expanded list of '25 Never Events' and, more recently, it has a updated the Never Events Policy Framework to provide greater clarity and recommended responses to these events. The document also contains data on the number and types of never events reported, revealing that 326 never events were reported to strategic health authorities in 2011–2012. This shows that there is a long way to go before the incidence of never events is brought down to zero.

Conclusion

The strengths and weaknesses of the metrics and indicators described in this chapter directly influence the success and failure of these initiatives. In addition to informing policy decisions, increasing public availability of performance metrics is guiding and empowering patients to make informed decisions regarding their health. This growing transparency in healthcare will play a significant role in driving quality improvement through greater accountability to public expectations and pay-for-performance incentives.

Root cause analysis

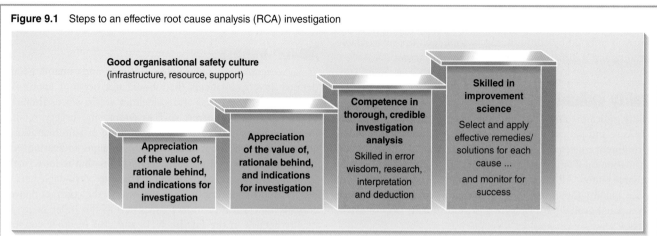

Figure 9.1 Steps to an effective root cause analysis (RCA) investigation

Good organisational safety culture
(infrastructure, resource, support)

Appreciation of the value of, rationale behind, and indications for investigation

Appreciation of the value of, rationale behind, and indications for investigation

Competence in thorough, credible investigation analysis
Skilled in error wisdom, research, interpretation and deduction

Skilled in improvement science
Select and apply effective remedies/ solutions for each cause ...
and monitor for success

Source: *NHS National Patient Safety Agency*

Figure 9.2 RCA investigation: fishbone diagram – tool

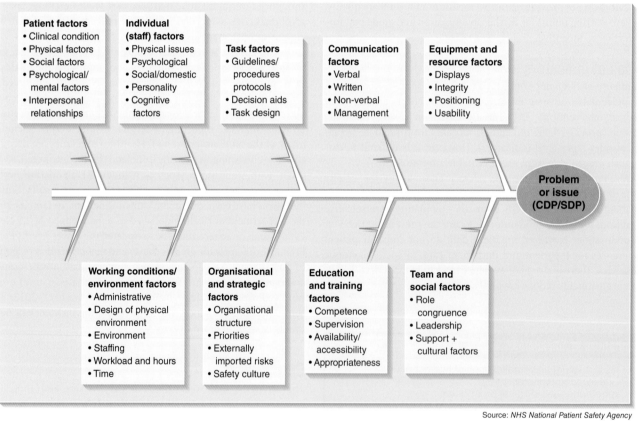

Patient factors
• Clinical condition
• Physical factors
• Social factors
• Psychological/ mental factors
• Interpersonal relationships

Individual (staff) factors
• Physical issues
• Psychological
• Social/domestic
• Personality
• Cognitive factors

Task factors
• Guidelines/ procedures protocols
• Decision aids
• Task design

Communication factors
• Verbal
• Written
• Non-verbal
• Management

Equipment and resource factors
• Displays
• Integrity
• Positioning
• Usability

Problem or issue (CDP/SDP)

Working conditions/ environment factors
• Administrative
• Design of physical environment
• Environment
• Staffing
• Workload and hours
• Time

Organisational and strategic factors
• Organisational structure
• Priorities
• Externally imported risks
• Safety culture

Education and training factors
• Competence
• Supervision
• Availability/ accessibility
• Appropriateness

Team and social factors
• Role congruence
• Leadership
• Support + cultural factors

Source: *NHS National Patient Safety Agency*

Patient Safety and Healthcare Improvement at a Glance, First Edition. Edited by Sukhmeet S. Panesar, Andrew Carson-Stevens, Sarah A. Salvilla and Aziz Sheikh
© 2014 John Wiley & Sons, Ltd. Published 2014 by John Wiley & Sons, Ltd.

What is root cause analysis?

Root cause analysis (RCA) is a method of incident investigation.

As such, it is a *diagnostic tool* rather than a safety solution in itself. RCA allows a systems approach (Chapter 26) to investigation and was selected as the methodology of choice by the National Patient Safety Agency when developing a framework for patient safety investigation in the NHS. The NHS approach aligns well with investigation methods used in healthcare and other high-risk industries across the globe.

Why investigate?

The primary aim of patient safety investigation is to learn from incidents and to determine what can be done to significantly reduce the likelihood of recurrence; the aim is *not* to apportion blame.

If, during an investigation, concerns of capability, recklessness or maliciousness arise, the Incident Decision Tree (IDT) should be used to provide guidance on whether and to whom these issues should be referred. Investigation and planned management of these particular concerns should not form part of the patient safety investigation process.

RCA process

• Investigations can be *comprehensive* or *concise* but must always include the basic elements to help ensure they are thorough, credible and actionable, and represent value for money
• Set clear terms of reference and follow them. Secure adequate time and skills, or record and report the impact of constraints
• Avoid lots of concise investigations. They can prove false economy

1 **Gathering and mapping the information**
   • You have to understand exactly what happened leading up to an incident before you can fully understand why it happened
   • Investigative interviewing should focus more on listening than on asking questions
   • Consult the patient and family as part of the investigation; they have a unique perspective and valuable information to share

2 **Identifying care and service delivery problems (CDPs and SDPs) – this stage involves identifying all the points at which:**
   • something happened that should not have happened; or
   • something that should have happened did not

3 **Analysing problems**
   • Using a fishbone diagram (or Ishikawa diagram or cause-and-effect diagram) as shown in Figure 9.2, place one CDP or SDP in the head of each fish (not the whole incident), then analyse why that course of action seemed the right thing to do at that time
   • A few carefully analysed 'fishbones' focusing on key CDPs and SDPs will deliver more benefit than many completed quickly
   • *Training* in *systems thinking* and *human factors* (including *error types* and *biases*) will aid impartiality and quality analysis
   • The *root causes* are the most significant contributory factors

4. **Generating recommendations and solutions**
   • Problems will rarely be resolved for the long term by applying discipline, training and updated procedures alone
   • *Training* in *improvement science* will assist with more effective selection and implementation of solutions

5. **Implementing solutions**
   • Amalgamate action plans from investigations. This encourages trend analysis and a more cohesive, high-level approach to resolving common issues
   • Avoid conducting more and more investigations with similar outcomes. Time must be allocated to implementing solutions and monitoring their efficacy

6. **Writing the Investigation Report**
   • Use an RCA investigation report template to facilitate trend analysis, audit and shared learning

Effective RCA investigation

The components for success in patient safety investigations are the same as those required for successful *clinical* investigations (Figure 9.1):

1 To avoid the extremes of delayed problem 'diagnosis' and resource wastage, triggers or indications for conducting an investigation must be correctly identified.

2 To obtain a good-quality, accurate picture of the problem, data gathering must be conducted by those skilled in the process.

3 The findings from the collection of data must be robustly interpreted and credible conclusions drawn by someone with analytical skills and an understanding of the 'anatomy, physiology and pathology' of the issue.

4 To ensure that improvement is achieved and measurable, expert selection, application and monitoring of effective treatment and remedial action are required.

5 If meaningful learning and improvement are expected from incident investigation, there must be organisation-wide support for this process.

Chapter 27 gives an example of a fishbone diagram in use.

10 Measuring safety culture

Introduction

'Safety culture' refers to the way that patient safety is thought about and implemented within an organisation. It is about the way safety is perceived, valued and prioritised. Safety climate is a subset of this, and refers to what staff think about safety. If an organisation has a 'strong safety culture', this means that processes are in place to keep people safe and that staff think that the organisation is doing a good job to promote safety.

The term 'safety culture' first became popular after the Chernobyl nuclear disaster, when people began suggesting that organisations could reduce safety incidents by developing a 'positive safety culture'. Safety culture has been measured in industries such as aviation, transport, manufacturing and oil and gas production. In healthcare, safety culture has become a key indicator over the past two decades.

The main components of safety culture include good leadership and teamwork, staff training, rules and safety processes, monitoring systems to identify and learn from incidents and communication and sharing to promote ongoing learning (see Figure 10.1).

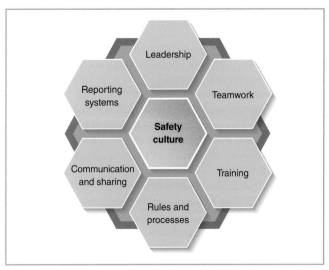

Figure 10.1 Key components of safety culture

Measuring safety culture

A number of tools are available to measure safety culture. Most involve surveys completed by managers and frontline staff. The most well-known tools are:

- Safety Attitudes Questionnaire
- Patient Safety Culture in Healthcare Organisations
- Hospital Survey on Patient Safety Culture
- Safety Climate Survey
- Manchester Patient Safety Framework

Many other surveys are also available (see Figure 10.2).

Usually the surveys used to measure safety culture are simple and quick to complete. They are designed to be completed regularly over time, such as once a year, to see if there have been any changes. Figure 10.3 provides an example of the format of one short safety culture survey.

Most tools are targeted towards hospitals, but a small number have been tested in other settings such as primary care, nursing homes and emergency services.

Box 10.1 describes a tool developed to measure safety culture in the United Kingdom. This tool is designed to be used in workshops with staff. Results are fed back and teams decide on changes to improve safety. The tool is then repeated after the changes are made – and the improvement cycle continues.

Some tools, such as the Safety Attitudes Questionnaire, have been more widely tested than others, but there is not enough evidence to say that one survey is any better or worse than others (see Table 10.1). In general, tools that are short, able to be repeated over time and able to be adapted for use in many different contexts may be most practical.

Much of the research about tools for measuring safety culture comes from the United States. We must be careful when transferring tools that work well in some countries to other countries where services are arranged differently. Similarly, tools that work well in hospitals might not be best for primary care, and surveys used in intensive care units or specialist wards might not necessarily be best for other services. When deciding which survey to use to measure safety culture, it is important to look at the tool carefully, test out whether it works on a small group and think about whether it is really relevant to the context you are working in.

Figure 10.2 Examples of the large number of tools available to measure safety culture

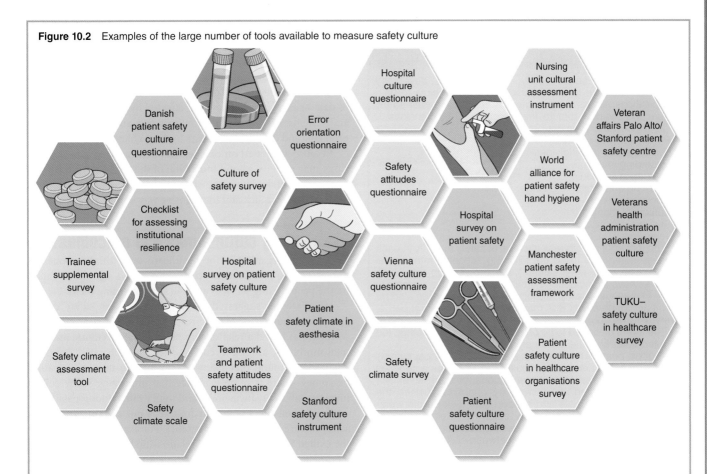

Figure 10.3 Example of the questions and format in one safety culture survey

A	B	C	D	E	X	
Disagree strongly	Disagree slightly	Neutral	Agree slighty	Agree strongly	Not applicable	
1.	The culture of this clinical area makes it easy to learn from the mistakes of others					A B C D E X
2.	Medical errors are handled appropriately in this clinical area					A B C D E X
3.	The senior leaders in my hospital listen to me and care about my concerns					A B C D E X
4.	The physician and nurse leaders in my area listen to me and care about my concerns					A B C D E X
5.	Leadership is driving us to be a safety-centred institution					A B C D E X
6.	My suggestions about safety would be acted upon if I expressed them to management					A B C D E X
7.	Management/leadership does not knowingly compromise safety concerns for productivity					A B C D E X
8.	I am encouraged by my colleagues to report any patient safety concerns I may have					A B C D E X
9.	I know the proper channels to direct questions regarding patient safety					A B C D E X
10.	I receive appropriate feedback about my performance					A B C D E X
11.	I would feel safe being treated here as a patient					A B C D E X
12.	Briefing personnel before the start of a shift (i.e. to plan for possible contingencies) is an important part of patient safety					A B C D E X
13.	Briefings are common here					A B C D E X
14.	I am satisfied with availability of clinical leadership (*please respond to all three*): **Physician**					A B C D E X
	Nursing					A B C D E X
	Pharmacy					A B C D E X
15.	This institution is doing more for patient safety now, than it did one year ago					A B C D E X
16.	I believe that most adverse events occur as a result of multiple system failures, and are not attributable to one individual's actions					A B C D E X
17.	The personnel in this clinical area take responsibility for patient safety					A B C D E X
18.	Personnel frequently disregard rules or guidelines that are established for this clinical area					A B C D E X
19.	Patient safety is constantly reinforced as the priority in this clinical area					A B C D E X

Box 10.1 Example of using the Manchester Patient Safety Framework

The Manchester Patient Safety Framework was developed based on literature reviews and expert input. It aims to help organisations assess their progress in developing their safety culture and see how 'mature' they are across 10 dimensions:

- Continuous improvement
- Priority given to safety
- System errors and individual responsibility
- Recording incidents
- Evaluating incidents
- Learning and effecting change
- Communication
- Personnel management
- Staff education
- Teamwork

The tool asks staff to rank the level of safety maturity in each of these categories using the following subsets: pathological ('Why waste our time on safety?'), reactive ('We do something when we have an incident'), bureaucratic ('We have systems in place to manage safety'), proactive ('We are always on alert for risks') and generative ('Risk management is an integral part of everything we do').

The tool is designed to be completed in a staff workshop led by a facilitator from the healthcare organisation.

A good point is that this tool can be used in hospitals as well as primary care, mental health and ambulance services and can be applied at an organisational or team level. For example, in England, 10 community pharmacies used the tool and 67 pharmacists and support staff took part in workshops to help assess the safety culture of their pharmacy. This helped raise awareness about patient safety and highlighted differences in perceptions between staff and areas for improvement.

This tool can be used to help teams reflect on safety culture, reveal any differences in attitudes between different types of staff and help understand what a more mature safety culture might look like. It has been used mainly in the United Kingdom, although some validation has taken place in North America.

Why measure safety culture?

Safety culture can be used to measure how well an organisation is doing in terms of patient safety. Other measures of patient safety such as error rates, death rates or record reviews can be difficult to measure consistently, be labour intensive regarding the collection of data or take a long time to be affected by changes in processes and systems. Measuring safety culture gets around some of these problems and can be an easy way to show changes over time.

Because it is based on people's views, measuring safety culture alone may not give a good indication of the levels of patient safety in an organisation. However, when used alongside other measures, it can provide a quick and inexpensive way of monitoring change.

Does safety culture improve outcomes?

The way an organisation or healthcare team thinks about and implements patient safety processes may have a significant impact on the people using services and the staff providing them.

Many studies suggest there is a link between safety culture and patient outcomes, but the relationship is not clear-cut. Some research has found a relationship between safety culture and hospital morbidity, adverse events and readmission rates. But other studies have found that safety culture has no impact on patient outcomes. There is more evidence that improving safety culture impacts staff safety behaviours and injury rates amongst staff.

Even when there is a clear link, it is not certain that a good safety culture creates better outcomes. For example, researchers in the United States examined the relationship between patient safety culture and rates of rehospitalisation within 30 days of discharge. Survey data from 36,375 staff from 67 hospitals were compared with risk-standardised hospital readmission rates. Poorer views of safety culture were associated with higher readmission rates for heart attacks and heart failure (Hansen LA, 2011). Other researchers in the United States examined whether safety culture was linked

---

Table 10.1 Features of the top five most well-known tools for measuring safety culture

Tool and developer	Where it has been used	Key strengths	Key weaknesses	Amount of evidence available
Hospital survey on patient safety culture *(AHRQ)*	• Hospitals in the UK, Belgium, China, Netherlands, Turkey, Saudi Arabia, Spain, Lebanon, etc.	• Can compare with other countries and industries	• Focuses only on hospitals • Has some validity issues	
Safety attitudes questionnaire *(developed from aviation tool)*	• Hospitals • ICU • Primary term care in many countries	• Well validated and established • Can compare with other countries and industries	• Not used much in UK • Some think it takes too much time to complete	
Manchester patient safety framework *(NPSA)*	• Hospitals in the in UK • Pharmacy in UK • Hospitals in Canada	• Focuses on a broader way of thinking about safety culture • Can be done in staff workshops	• Little has been published about usage	■
Safety climate survey *(University of Texas and IHI)*	• Hospitals in North America	• Short and easy to complete • Has been compared with other surveys	• Tested mainly in North America • Developed some time ago	■
Patient safety climate in healthcare organisations *(Stanford, funded by AHRQ)*	• Hospitals in the US	• Studies with large sample sizes have validated the tool	• Has been used mainly by one group of researchers • Tested almost exclusively in US hospitals	■

▨ = Sufficient evidence

■ = Limited evidence

with patient outcomes in intensive care units (ICUs). Data from 65,978 patients admitted to 30 ICUs were analysed and 2103 staff were surveyed. For every 10% decrease in safety culture, length of stay increased by 15% (Huang DT, 2010).

After initiatives are put in place to improve patient safety, there is sometimes a simultaneous improvement in both safety culture and patient outcomes. Therefore, rather than a one-way causal relationship where safety culture influences behaviours and clinical outcomes, there may be a circular relationship whereby changes in behaviours and outcomes also help to improve safety culture. If things are being done better, then staff might feel better about safety overall (see Figure 10.4).

Improving safety culture

An organisation with a positive safety culture encourages and retains learning, promotes open and honest reporting of safety incidents, does not penalise staff for systems errors, is prepared to identify its own shortcomings, rewards innovation and accepts constructive suggestions for continuous improvement. Improving safety culture is therefore about enhancing the entire way that patient safety is thought about and acted upon.

Organisations wanting to improve their safety culture may address key drivers such as:

- Ensuring leaders prioritise safety in policy and practice
- Visible participation by leaders such as ward walkrounds
- Having a standardised system-wide approach to safety
- Holding managers and staff accountable for safety
- Including safety in annual staff performance reviews
- Taking steps to minimise sources of error or harm
- Regular staff training about safety issues
- Asking staff, patients and families for improvement ideas
- Constant assessment of the safety significance of events
- Fair treatment of those who report safety incidents
- Recognising and rewarding good performance
- Sharing information about successes and improvement
- Listing safety incidents and successes on notice boards

A positive safety culture is established when safety is valued as highly as productivity or other outcomes.

The most important thing to remember is that the value of measuring and thinking about safety culture lies in raising the profile of patient safety and promoting conversations about safety.

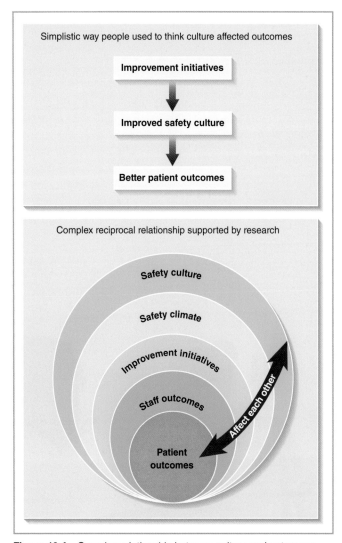

Figure 10.4 Complex relationship between culture and outcomes

The exact tools used may be less important than how feedback is collated and used. In other words, safety culture is about getting everyone on the same page in terms of improving safety – and this can have benefits for staff, for resource use and for patients and their families.

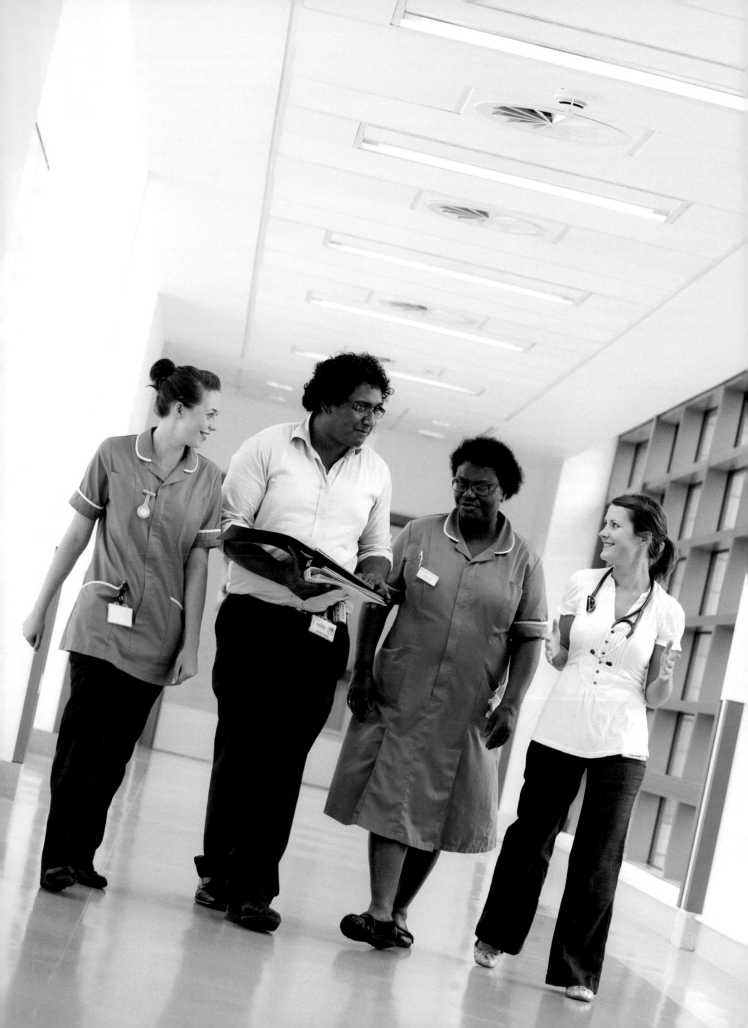

Risks to patient care

Part 3

Chapters

11 Medication errors

Figure 11.1 What are the different types of medication errors?

(a) Prescribing errors

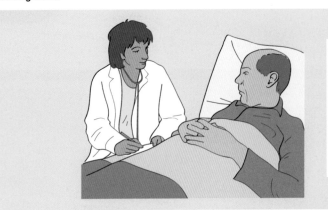

A prescribing error occurs when, as a result of a prescribing decision or prescription-writing process, there is an unintentional, significant: reduction in the probability of treatment being timely and effective, **or** increase in the risk of harm when compared to generally accepted practice. For example, prescribing an incorrect drug or dosage

(b) Transcription errors

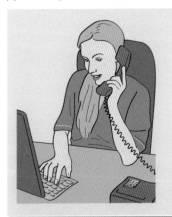

A transcription error is any deviation from the initial prescription or medication order, such as transcribing incorrect information regarding a patient's history

(c) Dispensing errors

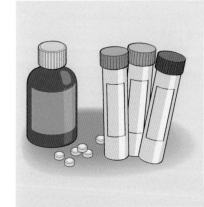

A dispensing error is any unintended deviation from an interpretable written prescription or medication order. Both content and labelling errors are included, such as dispensing an incorrect drug strength, form or quantity

(d) Administration errors

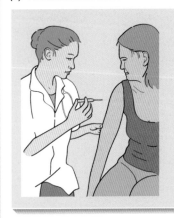

Errors that occur at the administration stage, such as failing to administer the right drug at the right time to the right patient

(e) Monitoring errors

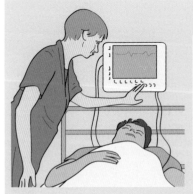

A monitoring error occurs when a prescribed medicine is not monitored in the way which would be considered acceptable in routine clinical practice. For example, failure to monitor for drug side effects

Patient Safety and Healthcare Improvement at a Glance, First Edition. Edited by Sukhmeet S. Panesar, Andrew Carson-Stevens, Sarah A. Salvilla and Aziz Sheikh
© 2014 John Wiley & Sons, Ltd. Published 2014 by John Wiley & Sons, Ltd.

Introduction

A medication error can be defined as any error that either resulted in, or had the potential to result in, an adverse drug event. Medication errors can occur at any stage of the medication use process, including the prescribing, transcribing, dispensing, administrating and monitoring of a drug. Not all medication errors have the potential to cause harm to the patient.

Box 11.1 The case of Wayne Jowett

Wayne Jowett, aged 18, was diagnosed with acute lymphoblastic leukaemia in June 1999. In June 2000 his disease was in remission and he entered the maintenance phase of his treatment. This consisted of the following drugs: 6-mercaptopurine (orally), methotrexate (orally), prednisolone (orally), vincristine (intravenously) and cytosine (intrathecally).

Wayne was scheduled to receive his chemotherapy drugs on the morning of 4 January 2001. On that day, the sister on the ward discovered that the chemotherapy drugs for Wayne were not prepared and asked Dr Musuka, Wayne's consultant, to prescribe them, which he did. The pharmacist prepared both cytosine and vincristine in the Sterile Production Unit. He had suggested that both drugs be administered one day apart to prevent an error from occurring. He then received a call from the ward to say that Wayne had arrived and so both drugs were sent together to the ward.

When Wayne arrived, the staff nurse, Ms Vallance, informed Dr Morton, a senior House officer, who was covering the ward. Dr Musuka was not informed. According to guidelines, intrathecal administration of chemotherapeutic agents should be supervised by a registrar. Therefore Dr Mulhem, the only registrar on the ward on that afternoon, was called to help Dr Morton. Staff nurse Vallance went to the Day Case unit refrigerator, where she found both chemotherapy items packed in one bag. She took the plastic bag to the treatment room and recalls saying: 'Here's Wayne's chemo'. Ms Vallance then left the room and the two doctors went on with the procedure. The lumbar puncture site was marked and local anaesthetic was infiltrated in the area. Dr Mulhem had a brief look at the prescription chart, but failed to recognise that vincristine was due to be given the following morning, nor that it should be given intravenously. Dr Morton performed the lumbar puncture. Dr Mulhem then read out aloud the name of the patient and the name and dose of the drug to be given. He did not mention the route of administration. Taking the syringe, Dr Morton asked whether the drug was 'cytosine' and Dr Mulhem confirmed that it was. Dr Morton then injected the contents of the syringe into Wayne's spine. Dr Mulhem then read out aloud the name and dose of the second drug (vincristine) and gave the syringe to Dr Morton. A few moments later, Dr Morton injected vincristine in Wayne's spine. Vincristine, when given intrathecally, causes central nervous system toxicity, producing progressive ascending myeloencephalopathy. A few minutes later, the two doctors realised that a serious mistake had happened and called for senior help.

Wayne Jowett suffered leg paralysis and respiratory failure. He was transferred to the ICU, where he was intubated and ventilated. His ventilator was switched off 4 weeks later. *Figure 11.2 outlines the failures in the case of Wayne Jowett using the Swiss cheese model.*

Adverse drug events (ADEs), or injuries due to drugs, are surprisingly common worldwide. At least 1.5 million preventable ADEs occur in the United States each year. The picture is no better in the United Kingdom, with approximately one in seven NHS hospital inpatients experiencing an adverse event, half of which were deemed possibly or definitely avoidable. For example, a patient with no history of allergic reactions, who experiences an allergic reaction to an antibiotic, has suffered an ADE. This ADE would not be attributable to error. However, an error would have occurred if a patient with a history of documented allergic reactions experiences an allergic reaction to a prescribed antibiotic because the medical record was unavailable or not consulted. Given the burden of ADEs, it is incumbent on all healthcare professionals to understand the types and causes of medication errors, to understand how often they cause harm and to help build safer medication systems.

Causes and potential prevention strategies for medication errors

Errors that cause harm can seldom be attributed to any one individual or factor. Many different aspects can contribute to an error, such as poor teamwork and communication, insufficient or missing information, illegibility, inadequate training, excessive workload, staff shortages, interruptions and distractions. The US Institute of Medicine (IOM) outlined a number of proven medication safety practices in *To Err Is Human: Building a Safer Healthcare System* to reduce errors in the medication process. These include:

• *Avoid reliance on memory and vigilance*: Work activities should be designed to minimise reliance on human short-term or long-term memory. It is unreasonable to expect individuals to remain vigilant for long periods of time. The wise use of protocols and electronic checklists at the point of decision making, for example, can assist physicians with repetitive tasks

• *Use of constraints and forcing functions*: This involves structuring critical tasks so as to guide users to the most appropriate action. Designing defaults for processes and devices like an infusion pump to default to shutoff (safe mode) rather than free flow can help prevent errors

• *Simplify key processes*: An effective means of reducing the likelihood of error is to simplify and standardise key processes. Examples of simplification include reducing the number of handoffs (e.g. multiple order and data entry) and the number of times a drug is administered per day

Health information technology

Electronic tools can help reduce the rate of errors and subsequent patient harm, such as:

1 Computerised physician order entry (CPOE) is the direct entry of medication orders into a computer system by a doctor or other authorised prescriber. At a minimum, a CPOE system can greatly reduce medication errors by ensuring orders are legible, complete and structured (i.e. they include a dose, route and frequency). CPOE is likely to be more effective at detecting and preventing errors when paired with other computerised systems, such as clinical decision support.

2 Clinical decision support (CDS) is computer software designed to assist doctors with decision making. These systems can provide clinical knowledge and guidance as well as patient-specific recommendations by matching patient characteristics (e.g. age and allergies) with rules in the computerised knowledge base. CDS systems can assist with the selection of drugs and dosages (alerts for drug–drug interactions and clinical guidelines), follow-up management (corollary orders and reminders for timely follow-up) and cost reductions (drug formulary guidelines).

3 Bar coding with an electronic medication administration system can substantially reduce transcription and administration errors, by alerting caregivers to potential errors before they occur. Scanning a patient's bar-coded wristband, for example, can verify the patient's identity; scanning the bar code of the item can double check that it is the intended drug.

4 Automated dispensing device (ADD) is a computerised drug storage device that allows medicines to be held and dispensed to a specific patient. These devices are more efficient at reducing medication errors if linked with bar coding and interfaced with hospital information systems. Unit-based cabinets can be placed in patient-care areas to help improve security and accountability for medications.

5 Smart intravenous infusion pumps or infusion devices with decision-support software can prevent errors by ensuring that the right infusion rate and duration are used. These devices can be programmed with standardised concentrations and infusion rates, so that a warning is triggered when settings are outside these established limits. The warning prompts the caregiver to reset the pump or override the alert.

Although health information technology (HIT) holds great promise to reduce medication errors, several studies have highlighted that unintended consequences associated with HIT implementation can occur with any implementation; for example, a research report observed an unexpected increase in mortality coincident after a commercial CPOE application was implemented. In this single-hospital study, it was reported how critically ill children had to physically arrive in the hospital and be fully registered into the system before order entry was allowed. Consequent delays in the administration of critical medication were reported, with fewer than half of the patients receiving antibiotics and vasoactive infusions within national guideline-recommended timelines. Although CPOE systems are still evolving, they are widely recognised as critical for reducing medication errors; ongoing assessment of systems integration and human–computer interface effects on clinical outcomes is essential.

National and international efforts to reduce medication errors

In the wake of the IOM report, the US Food and Drug Administration enhanced their efforts to reduce preventable harm by dedicating more resources to drug safety. The UK Department of Health also issued national guidance on the prevention of medication errors after a number of deaths were reported from the intrathecal injection of a Vinca alkaloid. In order to avoid such catastrophic clinical errors, the report recommended the use of non-Luer syringes, allowing intravenous administration of Vinca drugs only. These errors are amongst the most catastrophic; one tragic case is that of Wayne Jowett, as explained in Box 11.1.

In 2006, the World Health Organization launched the High 5s Project, an international collaboration aimed at addressing a number of key patient safety challenges in participating countries. This project facilitated the development and implementation of standardised operating protocols (SOPs) to prevent medication errors, one of which targeted the preparation, storage or administration of concentrated injectable medicines, such as concentrated potassium chloride solution, sodium heparin and injectable morphine preparations.

Conclusion

Medication errors are common and costly. Errors can be prevented by designing safety into the healthcare system. The use of HIT, such as CPOE, CDS, bar coding and smart pumps, can undoubtedly play a key role.

Figure 11.2 Swiss-cheese model outlining failures in the care of Wayne Jowett

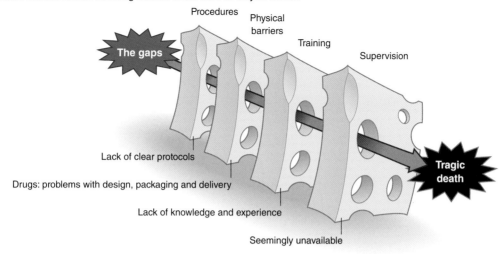

Lack of protocols

The protocol at the hospital stated that vincristine and cytosine should not be given on the same day, but on two consecutive days, to prevent any errors in their method of administration. Despite this guideline, and the fact that this was also noted by the pharmacist during the preparation of the drugs, these were sent together. The pharmacists dispatching them and the nurse receiving them did not question this, and staff nurse Vallance, who was helping with the lumbar puncture, also failed to notice it.

Drugs

Both drugs were packaged in separate boxes, but in one plastic envelope. They were also prescribed on the same prescription chart. In a number of hospitals, intrathecal chemotherapy is prescribed on a separate prescription chart, using a different colour from drugs administered intravenously. This would have alerted Dr Mulhem that only one drug was prescribed and should subsequently be administered. There is now a move to have separate Luer connectors for Vinka alkaloids which prevent wrong route administration.

Lack of knowledge and experience

Dr Morton had only been on the ward for 5 weeks and was still learning how things worked. That was his first oncology rotation and he had only administered intrathecal chemotherapy once before, under the supervision of his seniors. Dr Morton had not received any training regarding the intrathecal administration of chemotherapy agents. He assumed that Dr Mulhem was very experienced on chemotherapy and followed his advice without questioning it. However, this was Dr Mulhem's first job as a registrar. He had no experience with chemotherapy in the past. He had not received any training on chemotherapy.

Supervision: unavailable

The question remains as to where senior supervision occurred during this procedure.

12 Surgical errors

Figure 12.1 Surgery as a risky business

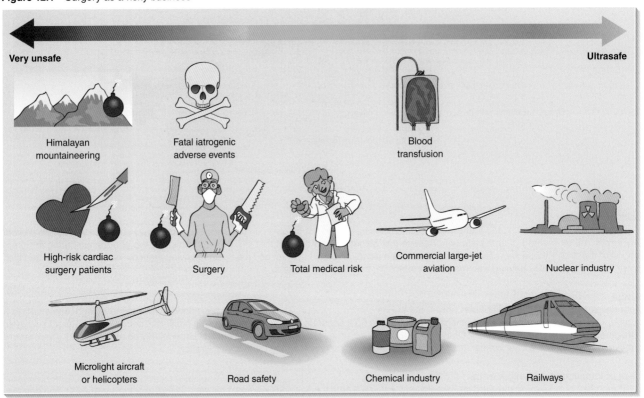

Source: Adapted from Amalberti (2005)

Figure 12.2 Surgical incidents reported to the National Patient Safety Agency from 2005 to 2008

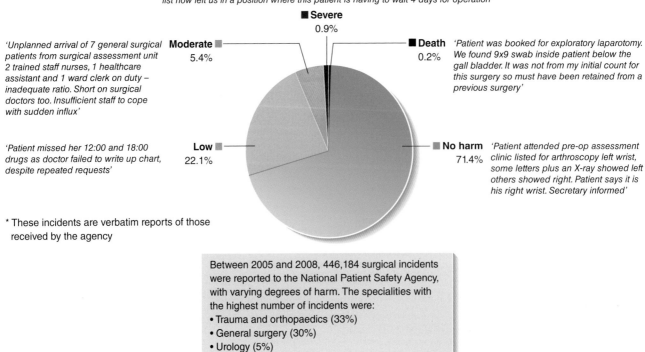

'Admitted on 15th with fractured neck of femur. High volume of trauma admitted this week. Additional list booked on Tues 16th to manage excess trauma. Cancellation of Wednesday list now left us in a position where this patient is having to wait 4 days for operation'

'Unplanned arrival of 7 general surgical patients from surgical assessment unit 2 trained staff nurses, 1 healthcare assistant and 1 ward clerk on duty – inadequate ratio. Short on surgical doctors too. Insufficient staff to cope with sudden influx'

'Patient missed her 12:00 and 18:00 drugs as doctor failed to write up chart, despite repeated requests'

'Patient was booked for exploratory laparotomy. We found 9x9 swab inside patient below the gall bladder. It was not from my initial count for this surgery so must have been retained from a previous surgery'

'Patient attended pre-op assessment clinic listed for arthroscopy left wrist, some letters plus an X-ray showed left others showed right. Patient says it is his right wrist. Secretary informed'

Severe 0.9%

Moderate 5.4%

Death 0.2%

Low 22.1%

No harm 71.4%

* These incidents are verbatim reports of those received by the agency

Between 2005 and 2008, 446,184 surgical incidents were reported to the National Patient Safety Agency, with varying degrees of harm. The specialities with the highest number of incidents were:
• Trauma and orthopaedics (33%)
• General surgery (30%)
• Urology (5%)

Patient Safety and Healthcare Improvement at a Glance, First Edition. Edited by Sukhmeet S. Panesar, Andrew Carson-Stevens, Sarah A. Salvilla and Aziz Sheikh
© 2014 John Wiley & Sons, Ltd. Published 2014 by John Wiley & Sons, Ltd.

Introduction

Advances in surgery have been made possible through extraordinary technological developments in delivering considerable benefits for patients. The increasing complexity of procedures, the number of professionals involved in the operating room and the complexity of the healthcare system have made it more difficult to deliver reliable and safer care. The number of patients who receive precisely the treatment expected could be better; whereas the number of patients who experience consequential errors is high. Other industries like aviation, nuclear and rail have managed to design extremely safe systems. Surgery has a long way to go (Figure 12.1).

Epidemiology of surgery

• 234 million surgical procedures are undertaken globally (of note, this is nearly double the annual number of childbirths worldwide)
• Eight million surgical operations are carried out every year in the United Kingdom
• Although death and complication rates after surgery are difficult to compare since the range of cases is so diverse, major morbidity complicates 3–16% of all inpatient surgical procedures in developed countries, with permanent disability or death rates of about 0.4–0.8%
• Almost seven million patients undergoing surgery have major complications and one million die during or immediately after surgery every year worldwide
• Nearly half of these surgical adverse events have been identified as preventable
• Figure 12.2 gives a flavour of the surgical incidents reported to a large patient safety reporting system

Technical versus non-technical skills

Technical skills include many different processes, including the recall of factual information, diagnosis and performing of practical procedures. Non-technical skills (human factors, discussed in chapter 5) are cognitive (e.g. decision making) and interpersonal (e.g. teamwork) skills. Analyses of adverse events in surgery indicate many underlying causes originating from behavioural or non-technical aspects of performance (e.g. poor communication between team members in the operating theatre) rather than a lack of technical expertise (most surgeons are good at operating).

Non-technical skills can be divided into four categories:
• *Communication and team working* – skills that ensure the transfer of information within and between clinicians and allied professional groups to maintain a shared knowledge and understanding of the patient (chapter 5)
• *Leadership* – guiding the team by providing direction, demonstrating high standards of clinical practice and care and being considerate about the needs of individual team members
• *Situation awareness* – developing and maintaining a dynamic awareness of the situation in theatre based on assembling data from the environment (patient, team, time, informational displays and equipment), understanding the impact of each environmental influence and anticipating what may happen next
• *Decision making* – utilising diagnostic skills for the situation and reaching a judgement in order to choose an appropriate course of action

Non-technical skills are as essential as technical skills when it comes to maintaining high levels of performance over a period of time.

Retained surgical materials

The economic impact of surgical complications relating to retention of surgical materials cost the UK taxpayer around £2 million per year, according to the NHS Litigation Authority (NHSLA). This traumatic experience is not limited to patients, but extends to their families. The human costs of short- and long-term follow-ups and the psychological implications are severe.

The incidence of retained swabs ranges from 1:9000 to 1:19,000 surgical procedures. Considering that 234 million surgical operations occur globally, such statistics are unacceptable. In most operating rooms, a system should exist to verify swab and instrument counts before and after surgery. However, most systems are labour intensive, and are perceived to interfere with surgery and other aspects of care, which may also be prone to error. Around one in eight operations involves at least one counting discrepancy, which increases the likelihood of a retained sponge and/or instrument. Sixty per cent of discrepancies detect a misplaced item, which would be categorised as a near miss. A recent 12-month analysis of all patient safety incidents reported to the UK National Patient Safety Agency's (NPSA) National Reporting and Learning System – the largest repository of medical errors in the world – revealed 496 incidents relating to retained surgical equipment in 5 years. The majority (94%) of those failures were fortunately prevented and corrected before any harm came to the patient.

The NPSA has taken a lead in identifying and monitoring reports of a national set of 'never events' for England and Wales. These events are serious and deemed to be completely preventable. One of the original eight 'never events' is *retained instrument postoperation*. Further work continues to develop technology to reduce human error, for example the development of bar-coded surgical sponges and surgical instruments, which are scanned by the nurses before being handed to the surgeon and vice versa.

Wrong-site surgery

Wrong-site or wrong-patient incidents are rare, but the consequences can result in considerable harm to the patient. It is often catastrophic for the patient (although perhaps less frequently fatal) and is a popular (and clearly delineated) error topic for reporting by mainstream media. The cause appears to be systemic predisposition. A recent study revealed 5940 cases of wrong-site surgery (2217 wrong-side surgical procedures and 3723 wrong-treatment or wrong-procedure errors) in 13 years. A particular interest has arisen in spinal- and neurosurgery, where wrong-site surgery occurs in between one in 4550 and one in 780 cases, depending on the procedure. Other factors such as fatigue, time pressure, changes to the operation, unusual patient anatomy and radiographic problems have all been identified as common risk factors. A one-year review of the database of errors housed at the NPSA revealed 353 cases of the wrong side marked on the theatre list. There were 150 cases of the wrong side marked on the consent form and 46 cases of wrong-side surgery (including some cases of burr holes and craniotomies being performed on the wrong side). Inclusion of wrong-site surgery as a *never event* (discussed in this chapter) and the use of checklists could help prevent this type of error.

Checklists

Checklists are not a new phenomenon and have been used regularly in high-risk industries such as oil mining, nuclear energy and aviation. In January 2007, the World Health Organization (WHO) began a programme aimed at improving the safety of surgical care globally. The initiative, called *Safe Surgery Saves Lives*, is aimed at identifying minimum standards of surgical care that can be universally applied across countries and settings. A core set of safety checks were identified in the form of a WHO Surgical Safety Checklist (Figure 12.3). It was designed to be used in any surgical setting and operating theatre environment. Each step on the checklist is simple, widely applicable and measurable, and it has already been demonstrated that its use can reduce death and major complications.

The checklist in England and Wales – a national perspective

In February 2009, the NPSA issued an alert requiring all hospitals in England and Wales to implement the WHO Surgical Safety Checklist by February 2010. One of the main drivers for success was the lead taken by the *Patient Safety First* campaign in England and the *1,000 Lives Campaign* in Wales in rolling out the checklist as part of their broader functions. These initiatives apply the principles of a social movement – *target individuals, engage on a personal level to inspire action and provide materials to make a difference locally, which can then be scaled up at a national level*. They created an inspirational movement that empowered frontline staff to bring about change. By April 2010, all hospitals had begun implementing the checklist using different approaches and with varying degrees of success. However, more than two-thirds reported that the checklist improved teamwork and safety, and almost 40% reported that they were able to capture more near-misses.

The task of implementing this simple life-saving tool has challenges:

• Negative clinician attitude and poor engagement ('I am a surgeon and do not make mistakes. Why should I be questioned by the nurse who is using the checklist?')
• Tendency to view the checklist as a mere tick-box exercise ('If I tick all the boxes haphazardly, I have done the checklist')
• Placing the checklist as a low priority ('We need to think about getting more theatre time and doing more operations')
• Lack of clinical leadership ('Surely, as surgeons and anaesthetists, we know what is best for the patients; does everyone in the team need to be counted as essential to patient care?')
• Poor acceptance of the strong evidence base of the checklist ('The checklist was assessed as part of a multi-centre study that involved some developing countries, so it cannot be that good for the UK')

• Poor implementation strategies ('The managers and clinicians have differing agendas')

A lean intervention – reducing surgical errors locally

The surgical emergency unit at the John Radcliffe Hospital is a 38-bed acute surgical ward in a teaching hospital in the United Kingdom. It receives all general surgical emergency admissions to the hospital. An audit of patient safety revealed that there was more than a 10% rate of harm experienced by patients on this ward due to deficiencies in compliance with recommended practice for important care processes – track and trigger tools (discussed in Chapter 16) were used in 77% of patients, and fluid balance charts were completed in 11% of patients. It was stipulated that a *lean intervention* (discussed in Chapters 26 and 27) could improve patient safety on the ward. Seven safety processes were selected, and elements of lean methodology were applied:

• Direct verbal communication between medical and nursing teams on daily rounds increased by 37% when visual aids and a sample protocol of individual roles were created
• Correct administration of prophylaxis for deep vein thrombosis (DVT) increased by 52% when a preprinted drug chart and self-audit were introduced
• Reduction of patients with drug-prescribing errors by 13% was achieved through prompt cards for commonly misprescribed drugs that were given to staff
• Use of alcohol gel for hand hygiene on entering ward increased by 8% as a result of better visual cues and more alcohol gel bottles being provided at convenient locations in the ward
• Correct use of venous site infection protocol increased by 33%
• Adequate monitoring of patients' vital signs and recording of their risk scores increased by 31% via a basic care checklist and a *track and trigger* tool (see Chapter 16) was implemented
• Adequate completion of fluid balance charts increased by 1% through no active intervention

Conclusion

Training in surgery focuses on technical skills. Whilst essential, this fails to recognise that surgeons cannot perform to the best of their technical ability unless they work in a well-functioning team (non-technical skills). Improved training in non-technical skills and use of tools such as the checklist can ensure that we practice safe surgery.

Figure 12.3 The WHO surgical safety checklist

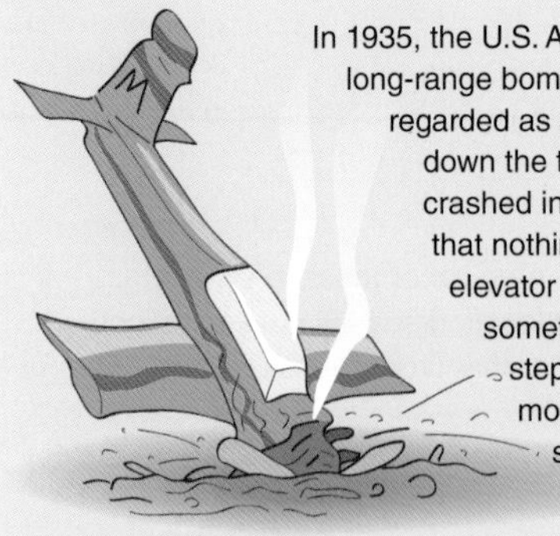

In 1935, the U.S. Army Air Corps held a flight competition for airplane manufacturers vying to build its next-generation long-range bomber. In early evaluations, the Boeing plane had trounced other designs. The flight "competition", was regarded as a mere formality. With the most technically gifted test pilot in the army on board, the plane roared down the tarmac, lifted off smoothly, and climbed sharply to 300 feet. Then it stalled, turned on one wing, and crashed in a fiery explosion. Two of the five crew members died, including the pilot. An investigation revealed that nothing mechanical had gone wrong. The pilot had forgotten to release the new locking mechanism on the elevator and rudder controls. A few months later, army pilots were convinced the plane could fly and invented something that would be used on the few planes that had been purchased.... A checklist, with step-by-step checks for takeoff, flight, landing, and taxiing. With the checklist in hand, the pilots went on to fly the model (B-17) a total of 1.8 million miles without one accident, and helped the US army launch its successful bombing campaign across Nazi Germany.

Surgical Safety Checklist (First edition)

Before induction of anaesthesia	Before skin incision	Before patient leaves operating room
Sign in	**Time out**	**Sign out**
☐ Patient has confirmed • Identity • Site • Procedure • Consent	☐ Confirm all team members have introduced themselves by name and role	Nurse verbally confirms with the team:
☐ Site marked /not applicable	☐ Surgeon, Anaesthesia professional and nurse verbally confirm • Patient • Site • Procedure	☐ The name of the procedure recorded
☐ Anaesthesia safety check completed		☐ That instrument, sponge and needle counts are correct (or not applicable)
☐ Pulse oximeter on patient and functioning	Anticipated critical events	☐ How the specimen is labelled (including patient name)
Does patient have a: **Known allergy?** ☐ No ☐ Yes	☐ Surgeon reviews: what are the critical or unexpected steps, operative duration, anticiptaed blood loss?	☐ Whether ther are any equipment problems to be addressed
Difficult airway/aspiration risk? ☐ No ☐ Yes, and equipment/assistance available	☐ Anaesthesia team reviews: are therw any patient-specific concerns?	☐ Surgeon, anaesthesia professional and nurse review the key concerns for recovery and management of this patient
Risk of >500mL blood loss (7mL/kg in children)? ☐ No ☐ Yes, and adequate intravenous access and fluids planned	☐ Nursing team reviews: has sterility (including indicator results) been confirmed? Are the equipment issues or any concerns?	
	Has antibiotic prophylaxis been given within the last 60 minutes? ☐ Yes ☐ Not applicable	
	Is essential imaging displayed? ☐ Yes ☐ Not applicable	

This checklist is not intended to be comprehensive. Additions and modifications to fit local practice are encouraged

The checklist outlines essential standards of surgical care and is designed to be a simple tool to improve surgical safety It consists of three key phases:

• **Sign in** – prior to anaesthesia ensures adequate preparation is made for any predictable difficulties and that the expected patient is about to receive anaesthesia

• **Time out** – just prior to incision is the final check that everything is in place for the procedure to take place in the safest environment possible. It is the final check that the right thing is about to be performed on the right patient, that everyone knows what the surgeon and anaesthetist are thinking or expecting, that the right equipment is available, that required imaging is displayed and that appropriate infection and venous thromboembolism prophylaxis is in place

• **Sign out** – ensures that the correct information will be given to recovery staff, that nothing is missing from the scrub trolley and that key specimens are correctly labelled

Source: Reproduced with permission of WHO

13 Diagnostic errors

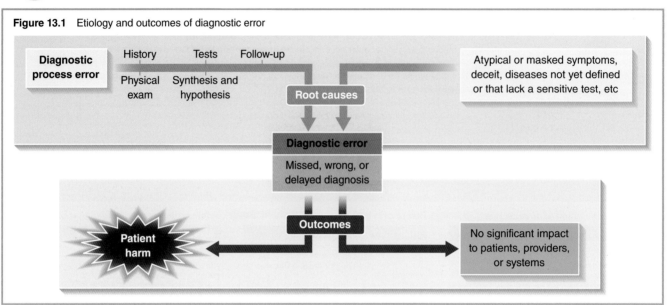

Figure 13.1 Etiology and outcomes of diagnostic error

Box 13.1 Case example of diagnostic error: wrong diagnosis of pneumonia

A 48-year-old male presented to A&E with cough, fever, hypoxemia, blood-tinged sputum, a tongue ulcer and an infiltrate on chest X-ray. The findings were attributed to community-acquired pneumonia. He was admitted to the intensive care unit (ICU) and started on broad-spectrum intravenous antibiotics. A Nephrology consultant was called to evaluate an elevated creatinine level and suggested the possibility of Wegener's granulomatosis. A sensitive and specific test for Wegener's was ordered (an anti-neutrophil cytoplasmic antibody, or ANCA, test). Five days later, the patient died of pulmonary haemorrhage and Wegener's granulomatosis was confirmed at autopsy. The ANCA test was never sent because it required a special form for 'send out' tests that was never completed, and the email the lab had sent to the ordering MD had never been read. Antibiotics are ineffective in treating Wegener's granulomatosis, but this often fatal disease responds well to immunosuppression.

Introduction

A diagnostic error describes situations in which the correct diagnosis is missed altogether, significantly delayed or simply wrong. Some of these situations are unavoidable, such as when the symptoms are masked or atypical, current tests lack sensitivity or the disease is at a very early stage. More typically, however, diagnostic errors reflect a preventable breakdown in one or more steps – cognitive, system-related or both – of the diagnostic process (Figure 13.1).

How do we arrive at a diagnosis?

Most diagnoses are made from the history and physical examination alone, and many errors can be avoided by paying special attention to these 'routine' aspects of patient evaluation. Other errors arise from problems with diagnostic testing, such as with performance, interpretation and follow-up of labs, imaging and other types of diagnostic test or procedures.

The synthesis or reasoning phase of the diagnostic process is especially important in deriving the correct diagnosis, and is the step most prone to cognitive errors. Clinical reasoning is often described by the 'dual process' paradigm (shown in Figure 13.2).

System I: When we encounter a new patient or a new problem, our brains instantaneously decide if the problem is recognised or not. Does it resemble something we have seen before, or something we learned during training? If the problem is recognised as something familiar, the diagnosis emerges effortlessly and quickly, based on our intuition, or what is more formally called 'System I'. System I is an automatic, subconscious thought process that typically works quite well. *In the case example in Box 13.1, the physician immediately recognised that the symptoms of cough, fever, hypoxemia and blood-tinged sputum were suggestive of pneumonia, which became the working diagnosis. Intuitive decisions work well for very common problems like pneumonia, but lead to errors when the real problem is something uncommon, like Wegener's granulomatosis.* True experts use intuitive, System I processing almost exclusively because they are so familiar with the content in their area. By definition, experts make the fewest mistakes, part of the reason that we trust intuitive decision making so strongly. Unfortunately, intuitive problem solving is

Patient Safety and Healthcare Improvement at a Glance, First Edition. Edited by Sukhmeet S. Panesar, Andrew Carson-Stevens, Sarah A. Salvilla and Aziz Sheikh.
© 2014 John Wiley & Sons, Ltd. Published 2014 by John Wiley & Sons, Ltd.

error-prone, especially if we are not experts. Intuitive processes are prone to a wide range of influences, both cognitive and emotional, that detract from reliable decision making. Some of the more common problems are detailed in Table 13.1.

Table 13.1: Common problems using System 1 (intuitive) problem solving

Jumping to a conclusion – Also called premature closure or satisficing, this refers to the tendency to accept the first reasonable solution that comes to mind and failing to consider alternatives.

Context errors – In trying to make sense of a new situation, the wrong context is envisioned. An example: Assuming the cause is gastrointestinal in a patient presenting with abdominal pain when the cause could be something else, such as shingles or referred pain.

Seeking confirmation only – This refers to the tendency to only look for evidence to confirm a diagnosis rather than looking for evidence to refute it, which may be more definitive.

Diagnostic inertia – Once established, a diagnostic label persists even if new evidence suggests some other possibility.

System II: If we do not recognise a pattern in the presenting symptoms, we revert to the tried-and-true method of solving puzzles – we apply deliberate, rational thought. Success in this effort will depend on our depth of knowledge, our ability to use evidence-based medicine and our skill in reasoning. This mode of problem solving, 'System II', is also error-prone, and it requires much more time, effort and attention than System I, but under normal circumstances it works. *In the case example, the physician should have realised that the elevated creatinine and tongue ulcer were not commonly associated with pneumonia. If the physician had switched to the analytical, or System II, mode of reasoning, this might have led to the consideration of other diagnostic possibilities, thus avoiding the diagnostic error that was made.*

All students start off using analytical reasoning (System II) exclusively, and as they gain knowledge and experience, more and more problems are solved using intuition (System I). When establishing a diagnosis, it is likely that some elements of System II will be at work; for example, when you reflect, at least briefly, on whether you are comfortable with the diagnosis or need to consider other possibilities.

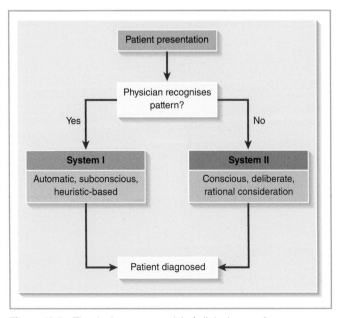

Figure 13.2 The dual-process model of clinical reasoning

How common are diagnostic errors?

Diagnostic errors are uncomfortably common. It is estimated that 40,000–80,000 preventable deaths occur from misdiagnoses each year in the United States. Furthermore, experts assert that 10–15% of *all* diagnoses are incorrect (with a small fraction leading to harm) and approximately 5% of people are misdiagnosed every year in the outpatient setting. Autopsy studies routinely find major diagnostic discrepancies in 20–30% of cases. Using chart reviews of discharged inpatients, the landmark Harvard Medical Practice Study identified adverse events in 7% of inpatients, and diagnostic mishaps were among the most common causes. Diagnostic errors generally make up the largest fraction of malpractice claims, result in the highest payments, and are the most difficult to defend in the court of law.

In addition to causing overt harm, diagnostic errors can lead to delayed, unnecessary or inappropriate testing and treatment. Besides the stress and concern of the involved patients, these cascades increase healthcare costs through problems with underuse, overuse and misuse of diagnostic testing strategies. Making the correct diagnosis, although complicated, is obviously critical to both obtaining optimal patient outcomes and using healthcare resources efficiently.

What factors contribute to diagnostic error?

The root causes of diagnostic errors include two categories that doctors or health systems can influence, system-related and cognitive factors, and a third category, 'no-fault' factors that are largely outside their control. These factors might operate synergistically, and typically multiple, contributory factors can be identified in a single case. System-related and cognitive contributions are identifiable in most diagnostic error cases, and 'no-fault' errors are less common (less than 10%) (Figure 13.3).

System-related contributory factors: refer to all the characteristics of the healthcare system and the operating environment that impact the safety and quality of care provided. Are there too many distractions? Is the workload balanced enough to provide each patient the attention they need? Are expertise, tests and equipment available when needed? Is care coordinated across sites and consultants? Are handoffs performed regularly and adequately? Is the staff well trained and engaged in their assigned work? Is the care process patient centred? Are trainees adequately supervised?

In the Wegener's granulomatosis case example, several system-related factors can be identified:
- *The lab required a complex administrative process for a test that should be performed expeditiously, and assumed that the staff they sent the message to read their emails regularly*
- *There was no process in place to ensure that critical tests were performed and reported on a timely basis. A process to 'close the loop' might have prevented this error by ensuring that the email was read and acted upon*

Cognitive-related contributory factors: largely fall within three categories: issues related to faulty knowledge, faulty data gathering and/or faulty synthesis. Faulty knowledge includes the physician lacking knowledge of a particular disease or the diagnostic skills to diagnose the current condition. Faulty data gathering involves incomplete gathering of the patient's history and examination, failure to order the appropriate tests or performing or interpreting diagnostic tests incorrectly. Faulty synthesis is by far the most common type of cognitive error, and reflects a failure in 'putting it all together'. The synthesis phase of diagnosis is especially prone to errors due to the many factors that detract from optimal cognitive performance. The intuitive diagnoses we derive using System I can be degraded by a wide range of problems, the most common of which are framing bias, context errors and premature closure.

System II errors commonly reflect inadequate knowledge about all the competing diagnostic possibilities, but can also go astray because of many other factors. Both System I and System II can be negatively impacted by stress, distractions, fatigue and affective issues, such as dealing with a relative or friend, or a patient who is disliked for some reason.

In the Wegener's granulomatosis case, several cognitive root causes can be suspected:

• *The physicians who initially evaluated the patient prematurely accepted the diagnosis of pneumonia because it seemed to explain the major findings, without considering other, more esoteric, possibilities in light of additional findings*

• *The ICU physicians who accepted the patient were influenced by the framing effects of the original ER diagnosis; they did not rethink the case on their own*

• *All of the treating physicians may have been biased by the presenting context. That is, the complaints of cough and the findings of infiltrate suggested a primary pulmonary etiology. In this case, the correct diagnosis of a primarily vascular process, Wegener's granulomatosis, may not have been considered because additional clues (tongue ulcer and creatinine) were not given adequate priority*

No-fault contributory factors: refer to root cause factors beyond the control of the clinician or the local standard healthcare system. This can include patient-related factors, such as when a patient fails to follow through with recommended diagnostic tests or follow-up appointments, or patients who are purposely misleading. Diseases that present atypically or at a very early stage, or findings that are non-specific, would also fall into this category. Another major category is situations where appropriate diagnostic tests are not yet available to assist in diagnosing a particular disease, but may evolve in the future. Similarly, some diseases can be diagnosed by exceedingly expensive or restricted tests that are not generally available in everyday practice.

How do we avoid diagnostic errors?

Diagnostic errors can be avoided by using a number of techniques. To begin with, this includes carrying out a thorough history and physical examination, and gathering all of the relevant background data. Be especially wary if the patient cannot communicate, or if someone else (the patient, another provider or the A&E doctor) suggested the diagnosis. Watch out for context and framing errors. It is worthwhile to spend a moment mentally reviewing some of the 'high-risk' situations (see Table 13.2) that predispose to diagnostic error.

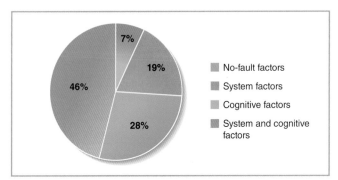

Figure 13.3 Contributors to diagnostic errors.

7%
19%
46%
28%

- No-fault factors
- System factors
- Cognitive factors
- System and cognitive factors

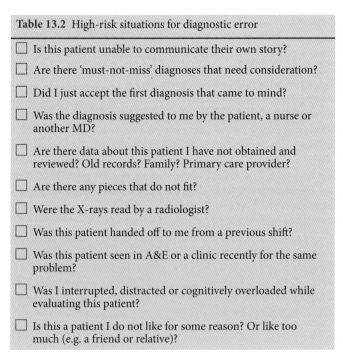

Table 13.2 High-risk situations for diagnostic error

☐ Is this patient unable to communicate their own story?

☐ Are there 'must-not-miss' diagnoses that need consideration?

☐ Did I just accept the first diagnosis that came to mind?

☐ Was the diagnosis suggested to me by the patient, a nurse or another MD?

☐ Are there data about this patient I have not obtained and reviewed? Old records? Family? Primary care provider?

☐ Are there any pieces that do not fit?

☐ Were the X-rays read by a radiologist?

☐ Was this patient handed off to me from a previous shift?

☐ Was this patient seen in A&E or a clinic recently for the same problem?

☐ Was I interrupted, distracted or cognitively overloaded while evaluating this patient?

☐ Is this a patient I do not like for some reason? Or like too much (e.g. a friend or relative)?

Cognitive-related interventions

When asked why they missed the correct diagnosis, the most common answer is 'I just did not think of it'. The best antidote to avoiding this problem is to invoke analytical (System II) reasoning. This involves taking a diagnostic 'time out' and pausing to reflect on how the diagnosis was established and whether it is trustworthy; thinking 'What else could this be?'; and trying to construct a differential diagnosis for every case seen, even if the patient already carries an assigned diagnosis.

Students can work towards increasing their knowledge and expertise, which in turn will improve clinical reasoning skills, by getting additional training and/or taking rotations in domains they are less familiar with.

Students must also never hesitate to ask for help. One can begin by soliciting second opinions from peers or other members of the team. Requesting consultation from a specialist is always warranted for cases one is unsure about. Having someone else think through the case independently is a powerful way to avoid diagnostic errors.

System-related interventions

Changes to the healthcare environment may also contribute to enhancing the reliability of the diagnostic process and preventing diagnostic error. Although such changes typically require actions and resources from more senior healthcare administrators, it is the responsibility of all frontline clinicians to bring opportunities for improvement to their attention.

Such changes may include improving clinical workflow, making sure training and supervision are appropriate, having specialist consultants available if needed and providing or enhancing medical hardware and software to support optimal diagnosis. Using a robust electronic medical record system with built-in decision support software can help to improve diagnoses in many ways. For example, the electronic record can improve communication and make it easier to order, find and follow test results. Electronic alerts can help avoid situations, like the Wegener's granulomatosis case example in Box 13.1, where essential test results have not yet returned.

Web-based decision support tools can be helpful in expanding the list of diagnostic considerations. A free online checklist to assist with differential diagnoses of common complaints is available at http://pie.med.utoronto.ca/DC/index.htm. Alternatively, simple tools like the VITAMIN CC&D mnemonic can bring other diagnostic possibilities to mind.

VITAMIN C C & D

V ascular
I nfection & intoxications
T rauma & toxins
A uto-immune
M etabolic
I diopathic & iatrogenic
N eoplastic
C ongenital
C onversion (psychiatric)
D egenerative

Changes in hospital policies and standard practices may also enhance the diagnostic process. For example, routinely following up with patients recently discharged from the hospital, or from an A&E visit, is a potential intervention that may reduce diagnostic errors and improve patient satisfaction at the same time.

Clinicians should also bring examples of diagnostic error to attention, so that they can be studied with the goal of helping avoid similar errors in the future. These exercises can lead to projects to redesign systems of care, and bring attention to cognitive issues as well. Finally, clinicians should always try to learn from their cases by requesting autopsies.

Involving patients

Patients should be partners in establishing the correct diagnosis, especially because they have the most at stake (Chapter 28). Clinicians should ensure that their patient knows how and when to get back to them if the symptoms change, or if they do not respond to treatment as the clinician thinks they should. Clinicians should always keep an open mind, be alert to findings that do not fit with the working diagnosis and remember that every diagnosis is just a probability, not a certainty.

14 Maternal and child health errors

Figure 14.1 The '3-delays' model

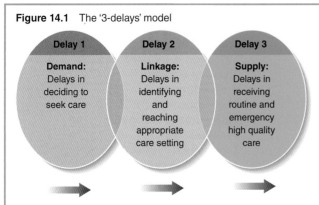

Delay 1	Delay 2	Delay 3
Demand: Delays in deciding to seek care	**Linkage:** Delays in identifying and reaching appropriate care setting	**Supply:** Delays in receiving routine and emergency high quality care

Figure 14.2 Linking communities to health facilities: roles and responsibilities of the task forces

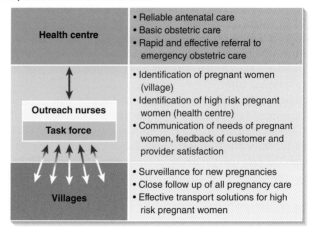

Health centre	• Reliable antenatal care • Basic obstetric care • Rapid and effective referral to emergency obstetric care
Outreach nurses **Task force**	• Identification of pregnant women (village) • Identification of high risk pregnant women (health centre) • Communication of needs of pregnant women, feedback of customer and provider satisfaction
Villages	• Surveillance for new pregnancies • Close follow up of all pregnancy care • Effective transport solutions for high risk pregnant women

Figure 14.3 The Institute for Healthcare Improvement's (IHI) Improving Perinatal Care driver diagram – a system perspective of patient safety

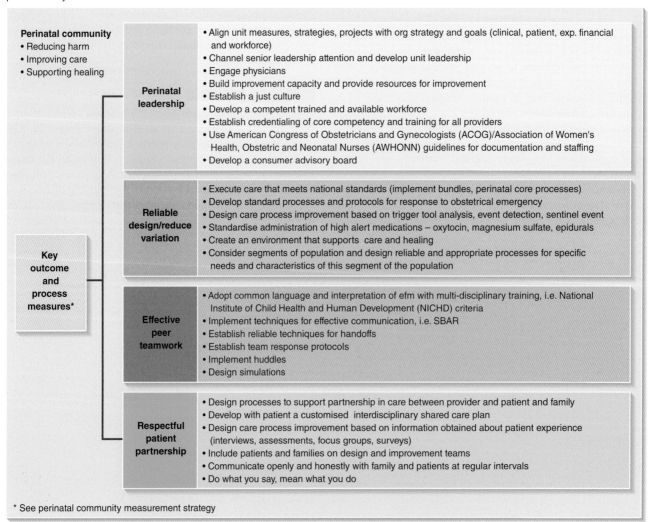

Perinatal community
• Reducing harm
• Improving care
• Supporting healing

Key outcome and process measures*

Perinatal leadership
• Align unit measures, strategies, projects with org strategy and goals (clinical, patient, exp. financial and workforce)
• Channel senior leadership attention and develop unit leadership
• Engage physicians
• Build improvement capacity and provide resources for improvement
• Establish a just culture
• Develop a competent trained and available workforce
• Establish credentialing of core competency and training for all providers
• Use American Congress of Obstetricians and Gynecologists (ACOG)/Association of Women's Health, Obstetric and Neonatal Nurses (AWHONN) guidelines for documentation and staffing
• Develop a consumer advisory board

Reliable design/reduce variation
• Execute care that meets national standards (implement bundles, perinatal core processes)
• Develop standard processes and protocols for response to obstetrical emergency
• Design care process improvement based on trigger tool analysis, event detection, sentinel event
• Standardise administration of high alert medications – oxytocin, magnesium sulfate, epidurals
• Create an environment that supports care and healing
• Consider segments of population and design reliable and appropriate processes for specific needs and characteristics of this segment of the population

Effective peer teamwork
• Adopt common language and interpretation of efm with multi-disciplinary training, i.e. National Institute of Child Health and Human Development (NICHD) criteria
• Implement techniques for effective communication, i.e. SBAR
• Establish reliable techniques for handoffs
• Establish team response protocols
• Implement huddles
• Design simulations

Respectful patient partnership
• Design processes to support partnership in care between provider and patient and family
• Develop with patient a customised interdisciplinary shared care plan
• Design care process improvement based on information obtained about patient experience (interviews, assessments, focus groups, surveys)
• Include patients and families on design and improvement teams
• Communicate openly and honestly with family and patients at regular intervals
• Do what you say, mean what you do

* See perinatal community measurement strategy

Patient Safety and Healthcare Improvement at a Glance, First Edition. Edited by Sukhmeet S. Panesar, Andrew Carson-Stevens, Sarah A. Salvilla and Aziz Sheikh
© 2014 John Wiley & Sons, Ltd. Published 2014 by John Wiley & Sons, Ltd.

Introduction

Because most high-income countries provide universal access to care, much of the focus on improving maternal outcomes in these countries has been on improving the reliability of safe obstetric care practices. In low- and middle-income countries (LMICs), a much broader effort is underway to tackle the enormous problem at hand: Africa continues to record rates of maternal death that were last seen in 'northern' countries over a century ago. For example, in 2010, the maternal death rate in high-income countries was 15/100,000, and in sub-Saharan Africa, the rate was 500/100,000 – a more than 30-fold difference. But progress in wealthy countries is not uniform; mortality rates can vary significantly depending on race and income levels. In the United States, the maternal mortality rate (MMR) among non-Hispanic black women (28.4/100,000) was roughly three times the rate of that among non-Hispanic white and Hispanic women overall (10.5 and 8.9/100,000, respectively).

In all countries, both the supply (reliability of delivered care) and the demand (community and patient) aspects of the system need to be addressed, as well as linkage structures to connect improved demand with more reliable supply. Major opportunities exist to ensure that knowledge of what works at all levels of the health system is transferred between these different settings. The '3-delays' model, a comprehensive approach to obstetric safety, has become popular as an organising framework for improving the care of pregnant women from the community to facilities (Figure 14.1). The model has informed work in Asia and Africa on improving decision making amongst pregnant women in Africa; the generation of novel community-facility structures that link pregnant mothers safely to the best place of care; and an adaptation of the Breakthrough Series quality improvement (QI) model (www.ihi.org), which is testing network thinking to inform a novel improvement team design that includes a web of players who are connected to a pregnant woman's journey to safe childbirth.

Delay 1: Demand

For many years, health systems have brought together pregnant women in high-income countries to educate and motivate good practice, and inform them of their options for safe and comfortable care during childbirth. While the social and educational benefits of these interactions are widely touted, the evidence of their effectiveness in improving decision making and safe outcomes is lacking. By contrast, community mobilisation through women's groups has been shown to be effective and cost-effective in changing care and care-seeking practices, and in reducing neonatal mortality in a range of settings in LMICs. The Women's Group intervention brings together women of childbearing age from a single village or group of small villages to undergo a structured, facilitated process of identifying, prioritising and deciding on an intervention to improve local needs, and then undertaking the intervention together. The typical journey from initial discussion to women-led intervention involves monthly meetings of the group over a 9-month period. A recent meta-analysis of women's groups in Asian and African countries has shown that these structures are associated with a significant decrease in both neonatal and maternal mortality. The exact mechanism of action that links women's groups to this decrease is not yet fully understood (Prost A 2013).

Delay 2: Linkage

Delay in reaching an appropriate and safe place of obstetric care is a significant determinant of poor obstetric outcomes in LMICs. Numerous studies have attributed a large portion (up to 73%) of preventable maternal deaths to issues related to failure of referral systems that ensure pregnant women receive the care they need, when they need it. While planning for women at high risk of obstetric complications requires particular attention, the value of over-reliance on stratification of pregnant women into 'high risk' and 'low risk' for obstetric complications has been questioned on the grounds that risk is hard to predict. Safe systems ensure that all women have easy access to reliable obstetric care, that unexpected emergencies can be promptly managed or referred and that high-risk women (Figure 14.2) are at an appropriate level of care at the start of labour. Innovative approaches that promote strong community facility linkages are being tested in countries with high rates of maternal mortality and unreliable access to care. In Malawi, health centres capable of basic obstetric care are being linked to communities through 'task forces' – committees, under the supervision of tribal authorities, which include village representatives and outreach nurses – that ensure safe passage to reliable antenatal and obstetric care for all pregnant women in the surrounding communities. In Ghana, referral and transport problems are being addressed through a novel adaptation of the Institute for Healthcare Improvement's learning networks. To ensure that community knowledge and inputs are maximised, the improvement team membership (which typically includes facility-based members) was expanded to include representatives of the community who have key roles in ensuring that pregnant women get to the right place at the right time to ensure safe outcomes. As such, the improvement teams included conventional care team members (midwives, doctors and clinic staff) as well as non-mainstream health purveyors (traditional healers, traditional birth attendants and chemical shop sellers), community leaders (spiritual and civic) and transport (taxi and ambulance) representatives. These improvement teams use the same QI principles (data-driven decision making, and testing of local ideas) as with more conventional QI projects to achieve their aims.

Delay 3: Supply

Improving the reliability of obstetric care has been key to efforts to improve safety and outcomes of childbirth. Using QI methods to improve the reliable delivery of evidence-based obstetric care is the basis of a number of successful interventions in high-, middle- and low-income countries. In Europe and North America, the perinatal collaboratives have brought together multiple hospitals and health systems around a set of concepts that provide the basis for systematic efforts to improve outcomes. The pace of improvement is accelerated when these healthcare units are networked, as this enables learning between sites.

After 2 years as an innovation community, IHI launched the IHI Improving Perinatal Care Collaborative in 2005 and it has continued since then. Over 150 hospitals and hospital systems in the United States and elsewhere have joined to focus on the reliable delivery of safe care to the obstetric patient in labour and delivery. The collaborative is designed with four main primary drivers: perinatal leadership, reliable design, effective teamwork and respectful patient partnership. The core theory, the Idealised Design of Perinatal Care, centres on a safety model of prevention, identification and mitigation which supports continuous quality improvement and having a system perspective (Figure 14.3).

The application of clinical bundles provides the infrastructure to the improvement methodology (Chapter 32). A care bundle is a set of evidence-based practices that improve patient outcomes when applied collectively and reliably. The actual measurement of these care bundles is what sets them apart from traditional measurement – the care bundle is measured as a whole, rather than measuring the individual components. This is termed 'all-or-none measurement'. As an example, if there are four accepted components that are necessary for appropriate care to occur, if one component of care is not delivered to the patient, the measurement is reported as 0%; the patient either gets all four (100%), or if any one is not completed the score is counted as zero (0%). This type of all-or-none measurement is a driver in changing the knowledge of a reliable delivery system of care.

Conclusion

Improving the safety and reliability of delivery of care is a journey and a process of continuous improvement. It involves changing the current paradigm of the system, which in many places remains hierarchical, to one that involves all stakeholders (providers, nurses, patients and families, administrators and communities) as necessary and needed change agents who function together as a team with one outcome in mind – to do no harm.

Slips, trips and falls

Figure 15.1 Multifactorial assessment and intervention

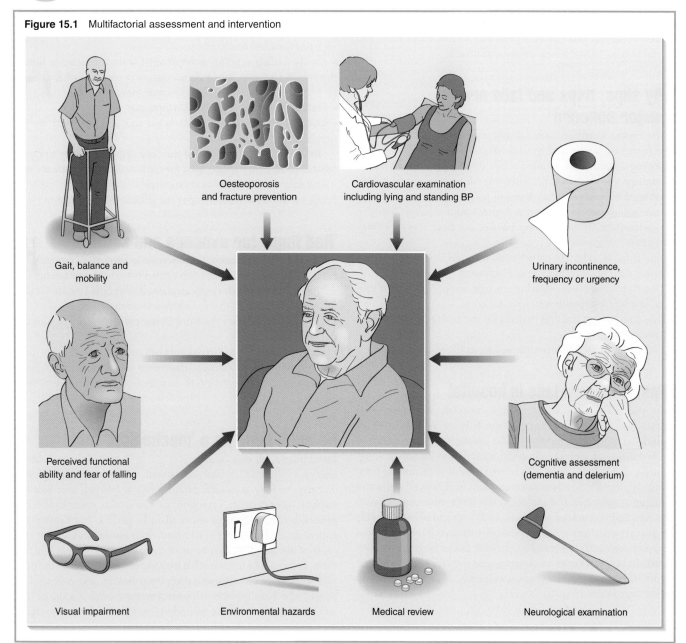

Gait, balance and mobility

Oesteoporosis and fracture prevention

Cardiovascular examination including lying and standing BP

Urinary incontinence, frequency or urgency

Perceived functional ability and fear of falling

Cognitive assessment (dementia and delerium)

Visual impairment

Environmental hazards

Medical review

Neurological examination

Patient Safety and Healthcare Improvement at a Glance, First Edition. Edited by Sukhmeet S. Panesar, Andrew Carson-Stevens, Sarah A. Salvilla and Aziz Sheikh
© 2014 John Wiley & Sons, Ltd. Published 2014 by John Wiley & Sons, Ltd.

Introduction

Falls are defined as: 'an event which results in a person coming to rest unintentionally on the ground or other lower level, with or without loss of consciousness'. Falls are a symptom of a number of interacting risk factors, not a disease, so when an older person seeks medical attention after a fall, there is an opportunity not only to prevent further falls and injury but also to reduce morbidity and mortality from treatable underlying conditions.

Why slips, trips and falls are a major concern

In the United Kingdom, over 1.5 million older people fall in their own homes each year, and around 300,000 osteoporotic fractures, including 75,000 hip fractures, occur. Risks increase with age; a third of people aged over 65 years will fall each year, and half of those aged 85 years will fall. Rates of falls for older people living in care homes can be three times higher than for people living in the community. These falls and injuries can have serious consequences:
• One-third of older people who fall will develop fear of falling, affecting their activity, lifestyle and wellbeing
• Two-thirds of patients with hip fracture do not regain their previous levels of independence
• One-third of hip fracture patients do not return to live in their own home
• Every 5 hours, an older person will die as the result of a fall

Slips, trips and falls in hospital

Many patients who fall are admitted to hospital – either for treatment of their injuries, or because the falls are symptoms of an underlying clinical condition. In the unfamiliar environment of the hospital, and with the effects of acute illness on top of long-standing illness, the risk of falls is even greater. Falls are the most commonly reported patient safety incident in almost all acute and community hospitals and mental health units, with over 280,000 falls reported in England and Wales each year and over 1,000 falls per year reported per acute hospital (of average size). Falls in hospital predominantly affect and harm older, frailer people; over 80% of falls in hospital occur in patients aged over 65 years, with the highest falls rates and the greatest vulnerability to injury seen in patients aged over 85 years.

Taking a falls history

As part of every admission for all patients aged over 65 years, and for younger patients with conditions that affect their mobility, routinely ask about any falls in the past year. Older people can be reluctant to admit falling, seeing falls as unimportant, or believing they could be seen as foolish or helpless. Phrasing the question as 'Any falls, faints or dizzy spells?' can help them to see that this is an important part of their medical history. If falls are reported, explore:
• Where did they fall? In their own home, or outdoors? What injuries? Have the falls left them fearful?
• When did they fall? Is there any pattern of time of day or repeated falls, or any recent increase in the frequency of falls?
• What were they doing? Were they walking, or had they just got up from their bed or chair?
• Do they recall slipping or tripping? Do they remember hitting the floor? Did they suffer from transient loss of consciousness (T-LOC)?
• Did they have any associated symptoms?
• Did anyone witness the fall? What did they see, and does it match the patient's account?

Ensure you have checked if they are cognitively able to give a reliable account of the fall. Even for cognitively intact patients, witnesses may be able either to corroborate or contradict the patient's recall, or may have noticed signs the patient was unaware of.

'Red flags' for syncope and seizure

Thirty per cent of blackouts in overs-65s present as unexplained falls. The patient should be investigated for syncope or seizure if:
• The fall is not convincingly explained or recalled (with T-LOC, the patient may say, 'I just found myself on the floor')
• The pattern of injury does not fit the patient's recall of how the fall occurred
• Facial injury – conscious patients will not normally fall face-first.
• They complain of dizziness, chest pain or palpitations

Remember that syncope is common (it affects up to 50% of people during their lifetime) and seizure is rare (around 1%)

No such thing as a 'mechanical' fall!

Describing a fall as a 'mechanical fall' is meaningless and almost always a failure of clinical assessment – unless you've had several days to fully assess the patient's vision, hearing, gait, balance, strength, coordination, cognition, cardiovascular, neurological and general health, and found them all to be perfect. Just because the patient describes a trip or slip hazard, don't assume this was the sole cause of the fall – they may be unaware of other risk factors affecting them, and could be unaware that they lost consciousness. In the unusual scenario of an otherwise completely healthy and independent patient who has slipped or tripped, describe the fall as a slip or trip, and be clear that they have no underlying gait or balance disorders.

Numerical risk assessment, or identifying and acting on risk factors?

Whilst some hospitals use numerical risk assessment scores to try to identify the patients most likely to fall, many tools in use have never had their predictive values tested, and even those scores that have been tested have poor predictive values; NICE Clinical Guideline 161 says risk scores should not be used. Given the frailty, age and illness of the majority of hospital patients, compounded by the effects of treatment and the unfamiliar environment, it can be better to simply consider all patients at risk unless they are independently and confidently mobile, and have no history of previous falls.

Multifactorial assessment and intervention

NICE Clinical Guideline 161 requires that all older people with recurrent falls, or who have fallen and have problems with gait and mobility, should be given an individualised multifactorial assessment and intervention – that is, a systematic process of identifying and, wherever possible, treating, modifying or better managing the older person's individual risk factors for falling. In a hospital, this will be provided by the multi-disciplinary team against a background of the general diagnosis and management of underlying disease. In addition to a falls history, an individualised multifactorial assessment and intervention must consider:

• gait, balance, mobility and muscle strength; perceived functional ability; and fear of falling
• visual impairment, especially recent changes in vision, visual field loss in patients with current or previous stroke, cataracts (early cataract extraction is of benefit in reducing falls risk), outdated glasses (if the frames look old, the lenses may be too) and difficulty managing bifocal or varifocal lenses
• cognitive impairment (including, in the hospital environment, assessment for delirium) and neurological examination
• urinary incontinence, frequency or urgency
• environmental safety (in hospital, this would include leaving personal possessions, drinks, call bells and mobility aids in reach; avoiding clutter; and acting on slip or trip hazards)
• cardiovascular examination, including lying and standing blood pressure to detect orthostatic hypotension
• medication review (see the 'Medication review' section for more detail) (Figure 15.1)

Medication review

Falls can be caused by almost any medication that acts on the brain or circulation, and reducing or discontinuing medication where the risks outweigh the benefits can help prevent falls. Key types of medication that increase falls risk include:

• Psychotropic drugs, especially benzodiazepines (but avoid abrupt discontinuation in habituated patients), antidepressants, medication used for psychosis and agitation, opiates, anti-epileptics, phenothiazines, sedating antihistamines and muscle relaxants
• Medication causing orthostatic or general hypotension, bradycardia, tachycardia or periods of asystole, including angiotensin-converting enzyme (ACE) inhibitors; alpha, beta and angiotensin II receptor blockers; thiazide and loop diuretics, antianginals and acetylcholinesterase inhibitors

In hospitals, medication-induced hypotension is a particular risk if previous doses of anti-hypertensives are prescribed to patients whose acute illness has resulted in their blood pressure dropping, as is 'compliance hypotension' (patients whose prescribed doses of anti-hypertensives do not reflect what they have actually been taking before admission).

Osteoporosis and fracture prevention

Whenever assessing for falls risk, bone health must also be considered. The most serious falls-related injuries are fractures, especially hip fractures. Patients who have sustained a prior fracture must have a bone health assessment and appropriate treatment in line with NICE Technology Appraisal Guidance 161.

After a fall in hospital

A National Patient Safety Agency Rapid Response Report identified that around 20% of patients who received serious injuries in a hospital fall had 'insult added to injury' through failures and delays in diagnosing and treating injuries from their fall. Following is some guidance on what to do after a fall:

• Don't become complacent – 99% of patients you see after an inpatient fall will not have serious injuries, but 1% will
• Stop, think and examine on the floor before allowing the patient to be moved – using a sling hoist on a fractured hip can be agonising, and using it on a fractured spine can be catastrophic
• Ensure any investigations or referrals for possible injury are treated with the urgency they deserve – the odds of recovering from serious injury are stacked against patients who were already acutely ill before they fell
• Consider pain relief, but be aware of the risk of masking symptoms
• Request neurological observations for any patient whose fall was unwitnessed – if no one saw the fall, you can't be sure they did not injure their head (even a cognitively intact patient could have retrograde amnesia from striking their head)
• Don't discontinue neurological observations too soon – especially in coagulopathic or anti-coagulated patients, in whom cerebral bleeds can take 24 to 48 hours or more to become symptomatic
• Always consider: 'Have they fallen because they are ill?' A fall in a hospital patient is often an ominous sign of deterioration in their condition, including potentially life-threatening infections, delirium or cardiovascular events
• Take the opportunity to prevent further falls – revisit multifactorial assessment and intervention

Final words

Getting old is inevitable, but falling in older age is not. The risk of falls and fractures in older people can be reduced, and it is the responsibility of us all.

Patient safety in paediatrics

Figure 16.1 National Institute for Health and Care Excellence (NICE) feverish illness in children guideline

The traffic light system: Children with fever and any of the symptoms or signs in the red column should be recognised as being at high risk.
Similarly, children with fever and any of the symptoms or signs in the amber column and none in the red column should be recognised as being at intermediate risk.
Children with symptoms and signs in the green column and none in the amber or red column are at low risk.

	Green – low risk	Amber – intermediate risk	Red – high risk
Colour	• Normal colour of skin lips and tongue	• Pallor reported by parent/carer	• Pale/mottled/ashen/blue
Activity	• Responds normally to social cues • Content/smiles • Stays awake or awakens quickly • Strong normal cry/not crying	• Not responding normally to social cues • Wakes only when prolonged stimulation • Decreased activity • No smile	• No response to social cues • Appears ill to a healthcare professional • Unable to rouse or if roused does not stay awake • Weak, high-pitched or continuous cry

Respiratory		• Nasal flaring
		• Tachypnoea:
		  – RR >50 breaths/minute age 6–12 months
		  – RR >40 breaths/minute age >12 months
		• Oxygen saturation ≤ 95% in air
		• Crackles
			• Grunting
			• Tachypnoea:
			  – RR >60 breaths/minute
			• Moderate or severe chest indrawing

Hydration	• Normal skin and eyes • Moist mucous membranes	• Dry mucous membrane • Poor feeding in infants • CRT ≥3 seconds • Reduced urine output	• Reduced skin turgor
Other	• None of the amber or red symptoms or signs	• Fewer for ≥5 days • Swelling of a limb or joint • Non-weight bearing/not using an extremity • A new lump >2 cm	• Age 0–3 months, temperature ≥38°C • Age 3–6 months, temperature ≥39°C • Non-blanching rash • Bulging fontanelle • Neck stiffness • Status epilepticus • Focal neurological signs • Focal seizures • Bile-stained vomiting

CRT = Capillary refill time, RR = Respiratory rate

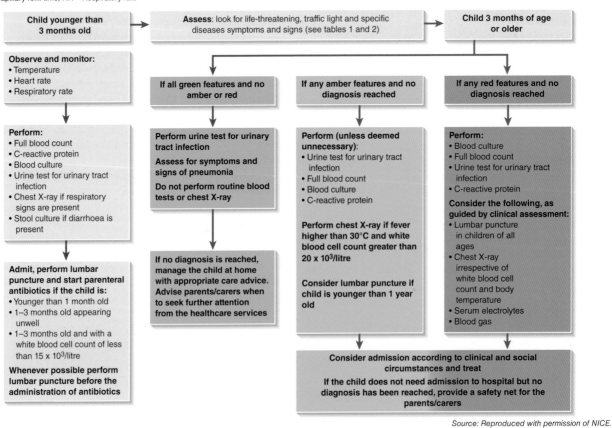

Source: Reproduced with permission of NICE.

Patient Safety and Healthcare Improvement at a Glance, First Edition. Edited by Sukhmeet S. Panesar, Andrew Carson-Stevens, Sarah A. Salvilla and Aziz Sheikh
© 2014 John Wiley & Sons, Ltd. Published 2014 by John Wiley & Sons, Ltd.

Introduction

The delivery of safe care to children is a major challenge for healthcare providers. Over the past 30 years, there have been major developments in medical science which have resulted in decreased mortality and better outcomes in all areas of paediatrics and child health. The aim now is for children to receive appropriate evidence-based care the first time, every time. This is the essence of providing highly reliable care to children, whether in the developed world or in less developed countries. The potential for this to happen in the less developed countries is great. Healthcare problems may differ, but in essence the principles are the same. This chapter outlines a few concepts essential to paediatric patient safety.

How safe is healthcare for children?

Since 1990, the global under-5 mortality rate has dropped from 87 deaths per 1000 live births in 1990, to 51 per 1000 in 2011. However, the majority are due to conditions that could be prevented or treated with access to simple, affordable interventions. Forty-three per cent of child deaths under the age of 5 take place during the neonatal period, so safe childbirth and effective neonatal care comprise an important focus. The key is the ability to deliver the care required to all children, whether this is immunisation, oral rehydration or safe water.

In the United Kingdom, the Confidential Enquiry into Maternal and Child Health (CEMACH) report *Why Children Die* found preventable factors in 26% of reviewed cases of child deaths, predominantly related to poor communication and non-recognition of the deteriorating child. A review by the former National Patient Safety Agency (NPSA) also identified difficulty in recognition as a key safety issue, as well as a high rate of reported medication errors, and the need for improved communication between healthcare professionals.

Why children are different

Patient safety is a young discipline, although it is central to healthcare. Paediatric patient safety is different. The expression 'Children are not little adults' is particularly true in medicine; children are different to adults in many ways. Table 16.1 shows key factors that influence risk.

Table 16.1 Factors that influence risk in paediatric patient safety

Difference in children	Impact on safety
Children go through different physiological stages.	Wrong equipment for different ages, or different medications
Drug dosing is weight dependent.	Medication error
Children suffer from different diseases.	Diagnostic delays
Children rely on adults and often cannot speak up for themselves.	Poor communication as a key factor
Often, children's healthcare is provided in adult-oriented facilities.	Lack of training and equipment, or mental health harm
Adult-trained health providers often provide care.	No knowledge of disease spectrum and changing needs, missed diagnoses and no detection of deterioration
Children are at particular risk from natural and economic stresses.	Less able to survive as margin of error is smaller than in adults

Definition of harm

There are technical definitions of harm, but often these mask the real issue of what happened to the child. The NHS Institute for Innovation and Improvement (NHS III) trigger tool prefers the definition 'Anything that one would not like to happen to oneself, one's own child or a member of one's family'. Using such a broad, personal definition helps us understand how pervasive harm can be. The key is that in patient safety, we want to reduce harm to the minimum, or eliminate it.

Variation in healthcare

Variation is evident throughout healthcare. We are all aware of patient characteristics that may explain some variation and differences in clinician capability. However, unwarranted clinical variation, defined by Wennberg as 'care that is not consistent with a patient's preference or related to [their] underlying illness', and variation in the way the system works are avoidable. Hollnagel defines 'patient safety' in terms of an organisation's ability to respond to changing conditions and carry out normal business without harming patients. Consider if, in a busy clinical department, there is an increased number of admissions and a member of staff is off sick. If safe, the unit would be able to manage to the same level of reliability and quality despite the stress under which it works. We all work in stressful environments where the predictable is regarded as unpredictable, and therefore crisis management is common. In less developed countries, if variation in delivery of simple interventions was decreased, millions of lives could be saved.

High reliability

The concept of high reliability comes from highly complex industries and environments such as aviation, nuclear power and space travel. It means that there is very little chance of things going wrong. Key features of high reliability described by Weick and Sutcliffe are:
• *Preoccupation with failure* – always asking what can go wrong before it does
• *Reluctance to simplify interpretation* – not simply blaming but trying to understand how the system and individual interact in harm
• *Sensitivity to operations* – always paying attention to what front-line staff and consumers of healthcare think and do
• *Commitment to resilience* – a learning environment continually adapting to change
• *Deference to expertise* – all decisions take into account the experience of patients and frontline staff who can often solve the problems that arise if given the authority to do so. The frontline staff (e.g. doctors in training) often know best how to solve problems and deliver safe care – we just need to make it easy for them to do it

Human factors

These refer to the interaction of humans and the environment in complex situations. The design of healthcare has only begun to understand the importance of this. To deliver healthcare is extremely complex, involving a number of steps that need to align. Design of the environment needs to anticipate how humans will act in these situations and how to avoid potential pitfalls (e.g. oxygen and air outlets with the same fitting). Simulation training with a focus on leadership and team communication is also essential for healthcare professionals to understand human factors and develop their skills. This can be simple and applicable in all settings.

Interventions to decrease harm
1. Decrease variation

Deming says that in order for the system to work to its optimum, it must reduce variation in how it delivers its outputs. In healthcare, this means standardise where possible, keep to policy to provide evidenced-based care and specialise only where necessary.

National Institute for Health and Care Excellence (NICE) guideline for feverish illness in children: a traffic light system

Feverish illness in young children is very common and usually indicates an underlying infection. It is a cause of concern for parents and carers. It is the second most common reason for a child being admitted to hospital and yet despite advances in healthcare in the United Kingdom, infections remain the leading cause of death in children under the age of 5 years. Fever in children can be a diagnostic challenge for healthcare professionals. It can be difficult to distinguish between a self-limiting viral illness and a more serious bacterial infection such as pneumonia or meningitis, especially when there is no apparent cause of fever, despite careful assessment. Due to a perceived need to improve the recognition, assessment and immediate treatment of feverish illnesses in children, the NICE feverish illness guideline was designed in 2007. The evidence-based guideline addresses the detection of fever, outlining suitable thermometers and the importance of taking parental reporting of fever seriously; management by remote assessment; and the traffic light system to predict the risk of serious illness (see Figure 16.1). The management of children with fever should be directed by the level of risk, as outlined in the guideline.

The implementation of guidelines, however, is poor. The use of improvement methods such as the Model for Improvement (see Chapter 23) is essential to achieve near-perfect compliance.

2. Detect harm

Traditional ways of detecting adverse events in paediatrics have relied on voluntary reporting. However, research has shown that only 10–20% of errors are ever reported and, of those, 90–95% cause no harm to patients. It is important to focus on harm, which targets the system, rather than on individual error.

Paediatric trigger tool

Structured case note reviews by medical and nursing teams on a regular basis help identify unintended harm within a service. By understanding the types of harm that may occur, the organisation can focus its improvement work on the areas of greatest impact and track improvements over time. The Model for Improvement and rapid test cycles were used by the NHS Institute for Innovation and Improvement to develop the UK paediatric trigger tool. Co-production was crucial for its design: decision makers, experts, service providers and users worked together to create a tool that worked for them all.

The tool measures adverse events in district general hospitals, acute teaching hospitals and specialist paediatric centres, with high sensitivity and specificity, through rapid (maximum 20 minutes) structured review of randomly selected case notes. Triggers listed in the tool are identified (e.g. INR >5), then a closer examination of the notes determines whether an adverse event has occurred (e.g. bleeding). If an adverse event has occurred and harm has resulted, then the category of harm is assigned. Figure 16.2 illustrates a page of the tool with examples of triggers and Figure 16.3 shows an early warning scores chart. The purpose of the review is to identify harm, not to discuss whether it was preventable. Trigger tools typically detect harm rates in excess of 30%.

3. Improve communication

In most clinical incidents, poor communication is an underlying problem. Handovers are an important part of clinical care and therefore need to be structured, consistent and reliable. The use of the SBAR (situation, background, assessment and recommendation) tool has become a fundamental part of safe care. All communication should follow an SBAR-type structure – both written and verbal (see Figure 16.2). Reading this back is an essential component to ensure that the information transmitted is accurate and understood.

4. Improve access to healthcare

Reducing newborn deaths globally: World Health Organization (WHO) safety tool to improve access to healthcare

The Millennium Development Goals (MDGs) were devised in the year 2000 to provide targets for improving social indicators around the world. MDGs 4 and 5 provide global targets for improving the health and survival of mothers and children. In September 2010, the UN Secretary General launched a re-energised Global Strategy for Women's and Children's Health due to concerns around reaching these goals by 2015.

WHO estimates that nearly four million newborns die each year globally within the first month of life; three-quarters of these deaths occur in the first week. Delayed recognition of early warning signs and delayed access to healthcare are the most common reasons for the majority of these deaths, which mostly occur in low-resource countries.

The Patients for Patient Safety team of WHO Patient Safety has created a patient-held safety tool that will help increase safety for both mothers and their newborn babies during the high-risk period: the first 7 days of life. Tool development was via a 'by patients, for patients' approach, ensuring it is easy to use by all mothers globally in settings of varying literacy. Based on a checklist concept, it contains safety checks for common danger signs for mothers and their babies to lead to more timely and appropriate accessing of healthcare.

5. Responding to deterioration

Early warning scores

Early warning scores are a means of identifying deterioration to prevent intensive care admission or cardiorespiratory arrest. This is especially important in children since it is well recognised that children who have died or required intensive care have shown signs of physiological or behavioural disturbance in the period prior to collapse. One of the CEMACH recommendations for paediatric care in the hospital was a 'standardised and rational monitoring system with embedded early identification systems for children developing critical illness'. An example of an early warning score is shown in Figure 16.2. There are important considerations to introducing early warning scores:

• Staff engagement is crucial. Recently, charts have incorporated nursing or parental concern as a score, recognising this importance
• The accurate completion of observations and calculation of scores are crucial, and so appropriate training of all staff is required
• The validity and impact of early warning scores are difficult to show, due to confounding factors such as rising standards of care and medical emergency response teams. Tibballs reviewed systems to prevent in-hospital arrest and found that the key feature is empowerment of any staff, however junior, and parents to summon help without deferring to senior colleagues or medical staff. Early warning scores may facilitate escalation of concerns using SBAR and therefore response to the deteriorating child

6. Decreasing medication harm

The prescribing of medications is not always performed with a high degree of reliability. A key factor to improving this is service redesign.

Zero-tolerance prescribing

At Great Ormond Street Hospital PICU, a programme of zero tolerance to errors has been instituted within a blame-free learning environment. Prescriptions can be written in designated no-interruption areas which are fully equipped with all the material required to prescribe. Immediate feedback on any errors found is given to ensure that there is real-time improvement. This has resulted in a substantial decrease in prescription errors.

Paediatric Emergency Drugs calculator app

Formulas for calculation of emergency drugs and infusions required for the resuscitation and stabilisation of the critically ill child are based on weight. This can lead to medication errors or delay in treatment while waiting for doses to be calculated.

The Paediatric Emergency Drugs app combines clinical experience from the Paediatric Intensive Care Unit of the Evelina Children's Hospital, Guy's and St Thomas' Trust, London, who have developed formulas and guidance for paediatric emergencies, with handheld technology developed by UBQO Limited. It is a simple and easy-to-use off-line application for both doctors and nurses on intensive care units and at hospitals stabilising and referring children. After entering the child's age, and weight if known, results of drug doses and over 80 infusions are quickly presented in a logical way. Physiological parameters based on the child's age are also presented to help recognise deterioration, with less reliance on memory of the normal age values of heart rate, blood pressure and respiratory rate.

Nolan describes system changes to reduce errors, acknowledging that many errors can be attributed to human cognition. He describes reducing complexity (e.g., availability of only paediatric concentrations of drugs), optimising information processing using automation and constraints (e.g. removing concentrated potassium solutions from children's wards) and mitigating unwanted effects of change (e.g. testing new equipment on a small scale with minimum risk). Drug calculators are an example of a system change to prevent human error. Dosing errors are consistently found to be the most common type of medication incident in children.

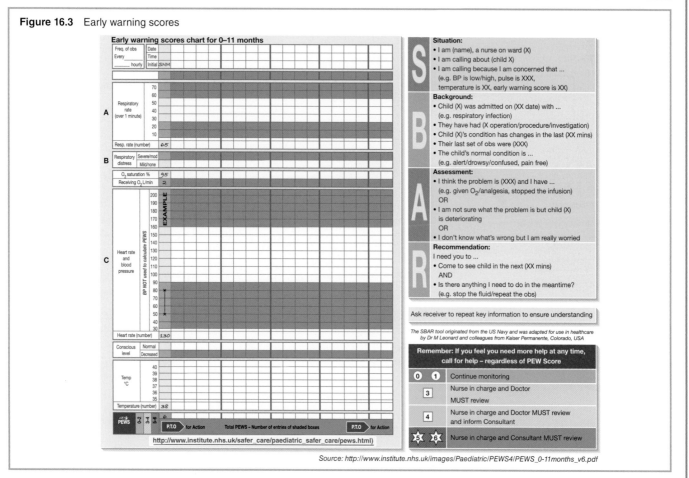

Figure 16.2 Paediatric trigger tool

Source: http://www.institute.nhs.uk/images//documents/SaferCare/Paediatrics/Paediatric%20Trigger%20Tool%20Form.pdf

Figure 16.3 Early warning scores

Source: http://www.institute.nhs.uk/images/Paediatric/PEWS4/PEWS_0-11months_v6.pdf

Technology in healthcare and e-iatrogenesis

Figure 17.1 Functions of information technology (IT) systems in healthcare

Informing and supporting decisions

Supporting patients/citizens

On-line information on health/lifestyle or illness/treatments

Tools for balancing risks/benefits/preferences to aid choices

Targeted educational interventions

Personal health records and self-management aids

On-line support networks

Supporting professionals

Case-specific diagnostic or treatment advice based on patient data and expert knowledge/evidence

Automated prompts and reminders for guidleline compliant prescribing, screening or reporting + safety alerts

Electronic guidelines, research reports and CME tools

Storing and managing data

Data

Patient-specific records, supporting care of individuals Population-based data, aiding research, policy and planning. Administrative data, aiding organisational and business processes. Integrated records, supporting mutiple stakeholders. Medical images

Records systems

Clinical (e.g. for capturing, displaying, sharing, linking or exchanging patient-specific data; or populating decision support)

Administrative (e.g. for audit, purchasing, billing, tracking service utilisation etc.)

Delivering expertise and care at a distance

Expertise and knowledge

Diagnostic or treatment advice from subject experts (e.g. telepathology)

Medical conferencing, clinical email

Mobile access to records; evidence; CDs

Care

Patient-provider email; internet consultations

Remote interventions (e.g. telepsychiatry, telesurgery)

Home and ambulatory disease monitoring and self-management support

Figure 17.2 Assumptions underlying the introduction of IT in healthcare

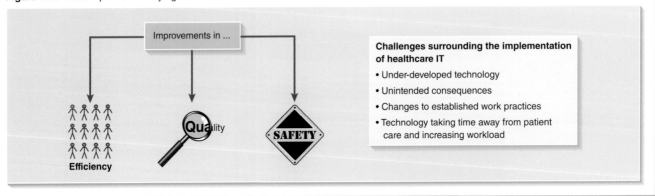

Improvements in ...

Efficiency

Quality

SAFETY

Challenges surrounding the implementation of healthcare IT

• Under-developed technology
• Unintended consequences
• Changes to established work practices
• Technology taking time away from patient care and increasing workload

Patient Safety and Healthcare Improvement at a Glance, First Edition. Edited by Sukhmeet S. Panesar, Andrew Carson-Stevens, Sarah A. Salvilla and Aziz Sheikh
© 2014 John Wiley & Sons, Ltd. Published 2014 by John Wiley & Sons, Ltd.

Introduction

Healthcare systems internationally are increasingly struggling to cope with demand due to increasing population sizes and demographic changes that are resulting in greater numbers of older people, who are often living with more than one long-term condition. There is an ever-increasing amount of medical knowledge and array of new treatment options. Healthcare providers and policy makers are therefore seeking out new and innovative ways to cope with these challenges. One key development in this respect is technological innovation, which has great potential to improve the quality, safety and efficiency of care (Figure 17.1 and Figure 17.2). Technology has the potential to reduce the risks associated with care provision by improving communication, promoting the accessibility of knowledge and assisting with decision making. However, technological tools may also introduce new risks. For example, they may prove disruptive to established working practices of users, and their introduction may inadvertently introduce new types of errors associated with their use.

Epidemiology of IT-related errors

• Healthcare technology is used by all healthcare professionals in developed countries, and is increasingly being used in developing countries
• Technical complications account for around 13% of adverse events in healthcare
• In the United Kingdom, around 400 patients a year die from adverse events related to medical devices
• Technology-related errors are expected to increase in line with new technological developments
• There is currently a lack of understanding around the measurement, analysis and categorisation of IT-related errors in healthcare settings

The nature of technology-related errors in healthcare settings

Errors and adverse events resulting from the use of technology are referred to as *e-iatrogenesis*. They most commonly occur in the following scenarios, and can involve both hardware and software:
• *The technology is needed but is unavailable for use*: Unavailability can result in users being unable to access and/or transmit data. For example, a review of medical notes and past medications may not be possible if the computer network is down or portable devices are not sufficiently charged. As a result, the user may not be alerted to potential drug allergies and contraindications, increasing the risk of inappropriate prescribing
• *The technology malfunctions during use*: This occurs if the technology is used as intended but the system does not perform the desired function correctly. For instance, a computer system may display incorrect information due to faulty algorithms, such as an X-ray result of another patient, potentially increasing risks of incorrect diagnoses
• *The technology is used in ways other than intended*: This scenario tends to occur if the use of the technology is viewed as too cumbersome and time-consuming by users in a busy healthcare environment. As a result, users take the quickest route to enter or access data in the system, which tends to compromise system reliability. For example, a user may find it easier to input data in free text boxes, but this can result in the inability of a system to pick up and alert users to potential adverse events such as contraindications
• *The technology interacts with other technology in unintended ways*: This can occur if essential information is not correctly transferred from one computer system to another. For example, a pharmacy system may fail to transfer important medication review-related information to the clinical ward system, resulting in the treating clinician not noticing a potential medication overdose

As can be seen, e-iatrogenesis can result not only from the design of the technology but also from the way it is implemented (or introduced) and used in individuals and organisations.

Design and implementation

There are several ways to mitigate against e-iatrogenesis. These relate to both improved technological design and implementation-related activities. We will discuss some examples relating to both aspects in this section.

Design

Technological systems should be designed with safety in mind and, in doing so, help users 'to do the right thing'. Such design features can help to address surrounding latent error-producing conditions as well as human cognitive shortcomings that may lead to adverse events. They are, however, not fool-proof and may bring their own inherent risks that users need to be aware of.

In relation to latent conditions, an example is bar-code verification technology which can help to reduce medicines administration errors and resulting adverse events by identifying the right patient and the right medication. This is accomplished by scanning a patient's wristband against the medication that is about to be administered, thereby minimising the risk of confusing patients and/or doses. However, although effective for some types of medications, such systems do have limitations. They can, for example, result in delays in administration if software access for immediate administration is required and the software is slow to load.

In relation to human cognition, an example is prescribing systems, which are commonly used to hold prescribing-related information and alert prescribers to potentially inappropriate doses, contraindications and allergies. However, the way information is displayed on the screen can significantly impact user behaviour. For example, the use of a large number of pop-up alerts may become tiring for users, resulting in them ignoring potentially important messages. This is commonly known as *alert fatigue*.

Usability analysis can help to minimise the potential for design-related errors. These can take a variety of forms, but the most commonly applied technique is *heuristic evaluation*. This involves assessment of a technological system based on an established set of usability indicators, including the following system features: the use of simple dialogue and language that are understandable for users, the ability to minimise users' memory load, consistency and provision of feedback to users, the ability to provide shortcuts and effective error messages and the capability to prevent errors and facilitate documentation.

Figure 17.3 The need for human-centred design

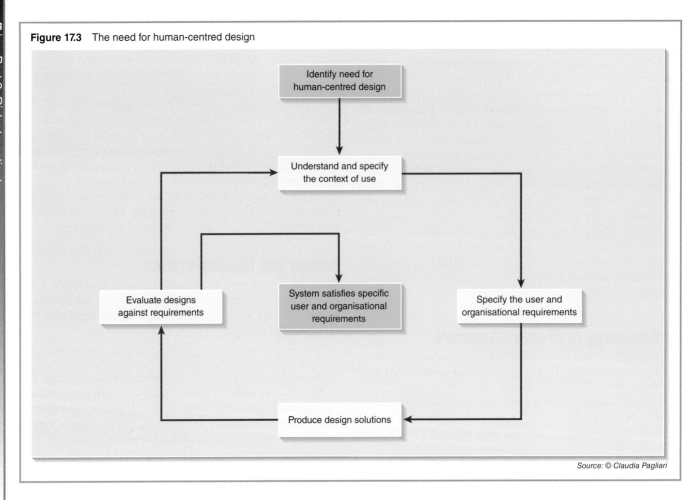

Source: © Claudia Pagliari

Implementation

In addition to design-related features, e-iatrogenesis can also result from the way that technology is introduced in organisations. For example, if users are not trained appropriately in how to use a technology, or if a system does not fit in with individual work practices, unintended patterns of usage may result. These are often conceptualised in the form of *workarounds*, or strategies employed by users to compensate for perceived inadequacies of the technological system. If, for instance, a system requires a large number of clicks for users to navigate it, they may choose to delay data entry activities until they find time later in the day. This in turn may result in records not being up-to-date and other healthcare professionals not being able to access important information. Potential mitigating strategies can include extensive work process mapping, involving the assessment of existing individual workflows with the technology, and re-designing processes involving the technology around these. This should involve extensive consultation of users and subsequent changes in technological design according to needs (Figure 17.3).

Initiatives to reduce technology-related errors

There are several initiatives that have attempted to reduce errors associated with technological systems in healthcare. These are mainly based on the design or implementation of best-practice guidelines and standards. We will outline a few examples in this section, but caution that the interrelated or iterative nature of design and implementation activities means that none of these should be viewed in isolation.

Safe implementation

Toolkits for local organisations implementing healthcare technologies aim to facilitate the process of change locally. These tend to guide implementers through the whole life cycle of introducing new technologies, from the conception of the project, planning, implementation and through to ongoing maintenance. One example is Stratis Health's Health Information Technology Toolkit for Critical Access and Small Hospitals (http://www.stratishealth.org/expertise/healthit/hospitals/htoolkit.html). Although based on the US context, many aspects of this work are transferable to organisations in other countries. Implementing organisations are provided with a range of resources that are adaptable to the particularities of individual contexts, including training resources and advice on work process mapping.

National guidelines

There are also increasingly design-related initiatives that aim to reduce errors associated with healthcare technologies; for example, in 2010, the United Kingdom's NPSA published guidelines for the safe on-screen display of medication information. These include advice for designers on displaying text and symbols, drug names, numbers and units of measurement and other information. A good example is the tendency of busy users to misread numbers due to trailing zeroes. So, if a system displays 'DOSE 5.0 mg', the user may in fact read '50 mg', resulting in an overdose. The NPSA recommends leaving trailing zeroes out, as a simple but effective mitigation against potential risks of overdoses (i.e. 'DOSE 5 mg'). This non-compulsory guidance is intended for the use of system developers (who may want to design their systems accordingly) and implementers (who may want to purchase systems that fulfil certain design-related safety standards).

A similar initiative is the NPSA's guide to the design of electronic infusion devices. This includes both hardware and software specifications and recommendations on how to address key safety concerns associated with these. For instance, some devices do not alert the user if the syringe and plunger are not adequately secured in the device, resulting in the potential for disengaging.

Safe implementation and design

There are also global initiatives targeting both implementation- and design-related sources of error. For instance, the World Health Organization's Department of Essential Health Technologies (part of the Global Initiative on Health Technologies) oversees international efforts to develop policies and guidelines for the use and implementation of healthcare technologies based on available empirical evidence. In doing so, the initiative has four sub-streams dealing with specific technological devices: Blood Transfusion Safety, Clinical Procedures, Diagnostic Imaging and Medical Devices, and Diagnostics and Laboratory Technology. Each member state is offered assistance in strengthening existing technologies within their economic capability.

Conclusion

Technological systems have made significant headway in ensuring that care is safer and more efficient. However, their use can introduce new sources of error and potentially avoidable harm. Several design- and implementation-related initiatives can help mitigate the risk of error, but technology should be viewed as a tool as opposed to a fool-proof mechanism to eliminate human cognitive and latent errors.

18 Nosocomial infections

Figure 18.1 Your 5 moments for hand hygiene

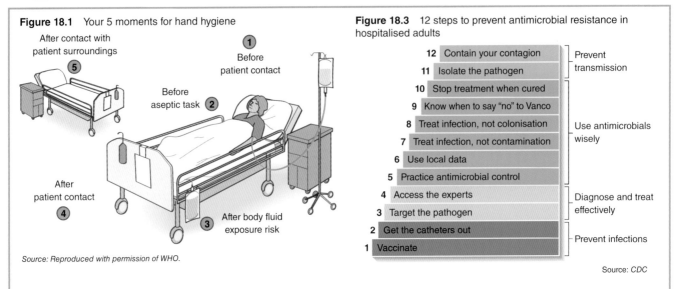

After contact with patient surroundings ⑤

① Before patient contact

② Before aseptic task

④ After patient contact

③ After body fluid exposure risk

Source: Reproduced with permission of WHO.

Figure 18.3 12 steps to prevent antimicrobial resistance in hospitalised adults

12	Contain your contagion	Prevent transmission
11	Isolate the pathogen	
10	Stop treatment when cured	Use antimicrobials wisely
9	Know when to say "no" to Vanco	
8	Treat infection, not colonisation	
7	Treat infection, not contamination	
6	Use local data	
5	Practice antimicrobial control	
4	Access the experts	Diagnose and treat effectively
3	Target the pathogen	
2	Get the catheters out	Prevent infections
1	Vaccinate	

Source: CDC

Figure 18.2 Surgical safety checklist

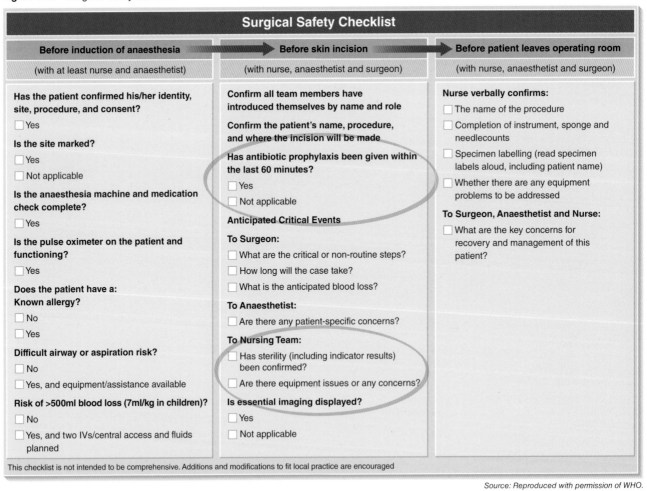

Surgical Safety Checklist

Before induction of anaesthesia
(with at least nurse and anaesthetist)

Has the patient confirmed his/her identity, site, procedure, and consent?
☐ Yes

Is the site marked?
☐ Yes
☐ Not applicable

Is the anaesthesia machine and medication check complete?
☐ Yes

Is the pulse oximeter on the patient and functioning?
☐ Yes

Does the patient have a: Known allergy?
☐ No
☐ Yes

Difficult airway or aspiration risk?
☐ No
☐ Yes, and equipment/assistance available

Risk of >500ml blood loss (7ml/kg in children)?
☐ No
☐ Yes, and two IVs/central access and fluids planned

Before skin incision
(with nurse, anaesthetist and surgeon)

Confirm all team members have introduced themselves by name and role

Confirm the patient's name, procedure, and where the incision will be made

Has antibiotic prophylaxis been given within the last 60 minutes?
☐ Yes
☐ Not applicable

Anticipated Critical Events

To Surgeon:
☐ What are the critical or non-routine steps?
☐ How long will the case take?
☐ What is the anticipated blood loss?

To Anaesthetist:
☐ Are there any patient-specific concerns?

To Nursing Team:
☐ Has sterility (including indicator results) been confirmed?
☐ Are there equipment issues or any concerns?

Is essential imaging displayed?
☐ Yes
☐ Not applicable

Before patient leaves operating room
(with nurse, anaesthetist and surgeon)

Nurse verbally confirms:
☐ The name of the procedure
☐ Completion of instrument, sponge and needlecounts
☐ Specimen labelling (read specimen labels aloud, including patient name)
☐ Whether there are any equipment problems to be addressed

To Surgeon, Anaesthetist and Nurse:
☐ What are the key concerns for recovery and management of this patient?

This checklist is not intended to be comprehensive. Additions and modifications to fit local practice are encouraged

Source: Reproduced with permission of WHO.

Patient Safety and Healthcare Improvement at a Glance, First Edition. Edited by Sukhmeet S. Panesar, Andrew Carson-Stevens, Sarah A. Salvilla and Aziz Sheikh
© 2014 John Wiley & Sons, Ltd. Published 2014 by John Wiley & Sons, Ltd.

Introduction

Nosocomial infection can be defined as an infection acquired in hospital by a patient who was admitted for a reason other than that infection. Typically the criteria for nosocomial infections are those occurring within 48 hours of hospital admission, 3 days post-discharge or 30 days of a surgical operation (e.g. an infection) following the insertion of an intravascular catheter (e.g. a central line). Whilst a central line is used to provide life-saving medications and effective monitoring, prolonged use almost inevitably leads to infection which can have significant consequences for the patient in terms of increased length of stay, treatment and, in a minority of cases, death.

Burden of nosocomial infections

The prevalence of healthcare-associated infections (HCAIs) varies between 3.5% and 12% in developed countries, and between 5.7% and 19.1% in developing countries.

In the United States, two million patients will acquire a nosocomial infection during their hospital stay, of which approximately 90,000 will die. The estimated economic burden is estimated between $28 and $45 billion. The vast majority of nosocomial infections, however, are preventable, and a large corpus of work has been undertaken globally to reduce them; some initiatives have demonstrated significant outcomes in reducing their prevalence.

Nosocomial infections are associated with increased morbidity and mortality, as well as increased admissions to, and length of stay in, intensive care, and the accompanying extra care costs from additional testing, drugs and procedures.

Case study

A 65-year-old man is admitted to hospital following a myocardial infarction, and required emergency cardiac surgery (a coronary artery bypass graft procedure). He made a good recovery over the first 48 hours on a surgical ward, and he is on target to be discharged on day 5. On the third day, he developed a fever with rigours, and the on-call doctor noticed an erythematous sternal wound with a serous discharge, and prescribed broad-spectrum antibiotics and intravenous fluids. The patient deteriorated further and was admitted to intensive care unit (ICU), where a Foundation Year 2 doctor inserted a central line and arterial line. He is diagnosed with sepsis secondary to a sternal wound infection.

The patient received additional antibiotics to treat a methicillin-resistant Staphylococcus aureus *(MRSA) infection over the next 4 days. By day 7 of his ICU stay, he is scheduled to return to the ward, when the ICU nurse records a low-grade fever. The ICU doctor examines the patient and notes erythema and pus at his 7-day-old central line insertion site. The doctor removes the central line and sends the tip to microbiology;* Staphylococcus epidermidis *is grown. The patient endures 2 further days of monitoring and antibiotics in ICU.*

In this case, the patient developed a surgical site infection (with MRSA) and a catheter-related infection. His scheduled discharge date was originally 5 days post-op, yet he stayed for a total of 14 days. His ICU admission was costly in terms of extra medications, multiple specimens and tests as well as bed blocking other patients from being admitted to ICU and being admitted for elective surgery. The patient became depressed following his prolonged ICU stay, and in the weeks following his hospital stay he was diagnosed with depression requiring antidepressant therapy.

Reducing HCAIs is not an easy task; its multifactorial nature makes it a difficult issue to contend with.

Initiatives to reduce nosocomial infections

In the 'Keystone ICU' project, funded by the Agency for Healthcare Research and Quality (AHRQ), 103 ICUs in Michigan, USA, participated in a state-wide safety initiative, which included instituting evidence-based preventive strategies for reducing CRBSIs (catheter-related bloodstream infections). The project focused on changing provider behaviour through addressing safety culture, incorporating a centralised education programme for team leaders at each institution and closely collaborating with infection control staff. The intervention almost eliminated CRBSIs in most ICUs over an 18-month follow-up period, and 1500 lives were saved. Following the Keystone ICU project in Michigan, 'Matching Michigan' was a national initiative seeking to emulate the success and involved over 97% of acute NHS trusts in England. The results were promising, and a 60% reduction in the number of CRBSIs was reported. However, on closer analysis of data, it was difficult to determine whether the reduction in CRBSIs resulted from the Matching Michigan project or from a coinciding nationwide drive to reduce nosocomial infections, since many trusts were already implementing part of the 5-point strategy employed in the Michigan intervention. There was also a decrease in other infections, which were not related to ICUs or CRBSIs.

The World Health Organization (WHO) has set up an international campaign called 'Clean Care Is Safer Care' which aims to promote the essential role of infection control in patient safety. 'SAVE LIVES: Clean Your Hands' was a campaign within this to promote good hand hygiene practices of healthcare workers (see Figure 18.1 for ways to help reduce the spread of potentially life-threatening infections in healthcare facilities). The WHO Surgical Safety Checklist also has elements in it (circled in Figure 18.2) which show the steps that need to occur to prevent nosocomial infections. The US Centers for Disease Control and Prevention (CDC) also has a 12-point checklist to prevent antimicrobial resistance (Figure 18.3).

There is a lot of important work being carried out to try to reduce nosocomial infections, but clearly more needs to be done. Understanding what nosocomial infections are, how they are acquired, what the repercussions and burden of them are and how they can be tackled are a critical part of any healthcare professional's clinical knowledge.

19 Mental health errors

Figure 19.1 Patient safety incidents reported between September 2010 and October 2010 based on care setting

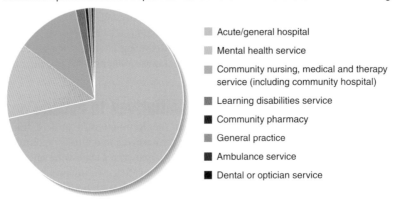

- Acute/general hospital
- Mental health service
- Community nursing, medical and therapy service (including community hospital)
- Learning disabilities service
- Community pharmacy
- General practice
- Ambulance service
- Dental or optician service

Figure 19.2 Types of incidents reported from mental health and learning disability settings within one calendar year (September 2010–October 2011)

Type of incident (with illustrative example)	Number of incidents
Patient accident – patient found on floor having fallen from bed	51,612
Disruptive, aggressive behaviour – patient verbally abusive towards staff	41,685
Self-harming behaviour – patient found to have inflicted a laceration to forearm using a broken CD	40,235
Access, admission, transfer or discharge (including missing patient) – delay in transferring patient to acute hospital for investigation of physical health problem	17,937
Medication – wrong medication administered	16,520
Other	13,704
Infrastructure (including staffing, facilities or environment) – not enough trained staff on ward to restrain a patient safely when required	3381
Documentation (including records and identification) – wrong patient details on medication chart	2386
Treatment and procedure – no physical health examination completed on admission	2101
Patient abuse (by staff and third party) – allegation of physical abuse by staff member towards patient	2242
Consent, communication and confidentiality – medication given without legal authority for detained patient	1651
Implementation of care and ongoing monitoring and review – patient not observed according to the level of observations agreed by the clinical team	1252
Infection control – outbreak of gastroenteritis on ward	504
Clinical assessment (including diagnosis, scans, tests and assessments) – patient not assessed prior to self-discharge	357
Medical device/equipment – resuscitation equipment not readily available	259

Patient Safety and Healthcare Improvement at a Glance, First Edition. Edited by Sukhmeet S. Panesar, Andrew Carson-Stevens, Sarah A. Salvilla and Aziz Sheikh
© 2014 John Wiley & Sons, Ltd. Published 2014 by John Wiley & Sons, Ltd.

Patient safety and risk in mental health

Safety is at the centre of all good healthcare service. It is particularly important in mental health, but is also challenging. Patient autonomy has to be considered alongside public safety. A good therapeutic relationship includes both empathic support and objective assessment of risk. Effective care includes an awareness of a person's overall needs as well as an awareness of the degree of risk that they may present to themselves or others. Risk management is a core component of mental healthcare. Assessing and managing risk are part of the daily work of mental health professionals.

Whereas significant strides have been made in understanding the burden of error and harm in hospital specialties, limited work has been undertaken in mental health patient safety. Quality improvement projects focused on safety are disproportionately focused on acute settings. Limited resources are dedicated to better understanding and working on safety issues within mental health or learning disability settings.

Patient safety incidents in mental health

The National Reporting and Learning System in England and Wales was introduced in Chapter 6; it is a database of patient safety incident reports. Figure 19.1 shows the proportion of all reported safety incidents that come from mental health or learning disabilities services.

In 2010, there were 193,165 incidents reported in mental health and learning disabilities services – with 165,988 (86%) of these from mental health and 27,177 (14%) from learning disabilities services.

Figure 19.2 shows a breakdown of incidents by severity of harm and type of incident.

The five most common types of reported patient safety incidents from mental health and learning disability settings:
* *Slips, trips and falls*
* *Disruptive and/or aggressive behaviour*
* *Self-harm* – including incidents of attempted suicide, completed suicide and non-suicidal self-harm
* *Access, admission, transfer and discharge* – including missing and absconding patients
* *Medication* – including dosage errors, wrong medication administration, allergy, adverse reactions and administration errors

Medication errors

Between October 2007 and September 2008, the NPSA received 7419 reports of medication errors involving mental health patients, representing 9% of all reported medication errors. Of these, 96% resulted in no harm, but there were 100 cases of death or severe harm. Around 92% of patients in contact with mental health services are prescribed medication, and it is highly likely that many incidents involving medication are going unreported. People with mental health problems may be particularly susceptible to medication errors due to various factors, including cognitive impairment, lack of insight into the nature of their mental disorder and need for treatment, or the complexity of mental health services and the number of different interfaces between primary care, secondary care, social care, community and inpatient teams.

In mental health and learning disabilities settings, medication errors with particular risks include:
* *Omission of medication* – for example, omission of methadone, anticonvulsant medication or clozapine can result in serious and rapid worsening of mental health conditions
* *Wrong dosing* – drugs such as lithium have a narrow therapeutic range, so a wrong dose could lead to serious medical complications and potentially death
* *Failure of monitoring* – drugs such as lithium or clozapine are subject to close monitoring. This is to prevent lithium toxicity or agranulocytosis for clozapine. A lithium-monitoring pack, similar to that used for oral anticoagulation therapy, has now been introduced which includes a patient-friendly information booklet, an alert card that patients should carry with them at all times and a record book to track critical information such as blood lithium levels and specific blood tests

Suicide and homicide

Suicide and homicide receive the most attention in mental health safety research, with comprehensive data sets and analysis conducted by the National Confidential Inquiry into Suicide and Homicide by People with Mental Illness.

Suicide

Approximately a quarter of all suicides are in individuals who have been in contact with mental health services during the 12 months prior to death (termed 'patient suicides'). The most common methods of suicide are hanging, strangulation and self-poisoning (overdose). The National Confidential Inquiry has been collecting and studying data on patient suicides in the United Kingdom since 1997. Analysis of this large national data set has allowed the implementation of national suicide prevention strategies, with the first of these dating back to 2001 ('12 Points to a Safer Service'). Recommendations included:
* The removal of ligature points on wards
* Follow-up within 7 days of discharge for all patient with severe mental illness or a history of self-harm within the last 3 months
* Patients with a history of self-harm to receive no more than 2 weeks' medication at a time
* Development of assertive outreach teams to prevent loss of contact with vulnerable and high-risk individuals
* 24-hour crisis teams in the community

The development of an evidence-based suicide prevention strategy with clear clinical recommendations and prominence in national policy has led to reductions in the numbers of patient suicides. From 2000, there was a 62% fall in the number of inpatients dying by suicide, and a 54% fall in the number dying by hanging. In addition to national strategies, there have been tools developed to support local services in assuring best practice on suicide prevention. These include the Suicide Prevention Toolkits for mental health services, primary care, urgent settings and ambulance services, which provide audit tools and dashboards to monitor performance on areas that are core to reducing the risk of suicide. In 2012, a new cross-government suicide prevention strategy for England broadened the focus from patient suicides to reducing the suicide rate in the general population, with the impetus on reducing

Figure 19.3 The seven steps to improving patient safety in mental health

Step 1	**Build a safety culture**
	• Create a culture that is open and fair
	• Staff should have a constant and active awareness of the potential for things to go wrong
	• Staff and the organisation should be able to acknowledge mistakes, learn from them and take action to put things right
	• Information should be shared freely and openly with service users when things go wrong

Step 2	**Lead and support your staff**
	• Strong leadership with clear policies in relation to safety and a willingness to implement best practice at service level
	• Leaders should be visible and active in leading patient safety initiatives

Step 3	**Integrate your risk management activity**
	• Patient safety is a key component of risk management, and should be integrated with staff safety, complaints management, litigation and claims handling, and financial and environmental risk
	• The risk management system should be supported by a risk management strategy (involving a consistent approach to training, management, analysis and investigation of all risks), a programme of proactive risk assessments and the compilation of an organisation-wide risk register

Step 4	**Strengthen reporting in mental healthcare**
	• A high level of reporting within an organisation indicates a better safety culture: the more aware staff are of safety problems, the more likely they are to report
	• Key to improving reporting is ensuring that learning from the reports received are widely disseminated and then acted upon

Step 5	**Involve and communicate with service users and the public**
	• Involving service users and the public in developing safer services at a strategic level
	• Involving service users in their own care and treatment
	• Encouraging an open, two-way dialogue between health professionals and service users when things go wrong

Step 6	**Learn and share safety lessons**
	• Look at the underlying causes of patient safety incidents and learn how to prevent them from happening again
	• Use Root Cause Analysis, and consider aggregating investigations to improve safety through addressing common issues

Step 7	**Implement solutions to prevent harm**
	• Solutions need to be simple to implement and low cost
	• Solutions range from designing out the potential for harm, designing systems which make it easy for people to do the right thing, to raising awareness and understanding

the risk of suicide in key high-risk groups, tailoring approaches to improve mental health in specific groups, reducing access to the means of suicide and providing better information and support to those bereaved or affected by suicide.

Homicide

When a homicide occurs involving a patient with mental illness, there is significant media and political interest. Mandatory independent homicide inquiries were introduced in England in 1994, but there has been much criticism of the value of these investigations in improving safety in mental healthcare. The common preconception, often fostered by the media, is that people with a mental health problem are dangerous. It is tempting to think that finding ways of treating the mental illness will eliminate risk and prevent the homicides from occurring. However, it is estimated that 21% of the homicides committed by people with mental illness were preventable by mental health services. Recent evidence suggests that although schizophrenia and other psychoses are associated with violence and violent offending, particularly homicide, most of this excess risk appears to be mediated by substance abuse comorbidity.

The number of homicides committed by people with a mental health problem has increased from 54 homicides in 1997 to 77 in 2005. The proportion of these committed by individuals with a psychotic disorder at the time of the offence rose from 41% in 1997 to 62% in 2005. Of all those convicted of a homicide between 1997 and 2005, approximately 10% had been in contact with mental health services in the previous year. Recent evidence suggests that this upward trend in patient homicides has now reversed, following a peak in 2006.

Independent inquiries after homicides have found a number of recurring themes, which should therefore be priorities for safety improvement work within mental health services. These include inadequate risk assessment and management, poor communication between professional agencies, inadequate application of the Care Programme Approach, insufficient response to the patient's non-engagement, failure to use the Mental Health Act appropriately, failing to listen to carers and non-compliance with medication.

Physical health monitoring

Physical health and mental health are inextricably linked. Mental illness is associated with increased risk of physical illness, arising in part from a less healthy lifestyle and more frequent health-risk behaviours. Conversely, physical illness increases the risk of mental illness. For example, depression is associated with 67% increased mortality from cardiovascular disease, 50% increased mortality from cancer, twofold increased mortality from respiratory disease and threefold increased mortality from metabolic disease. Rates of depression are double in those with diabetes, hypertension, coronary artery disease and heart failure, and triple in those with end-stage renal failure, chronic obstructive pulmonary disease and cerebrovascular disease. People with schizophrenia and bipolar disorder die on average 25 years earlier than the general population, largely because of physical health problems. Schizophrenia is associated with increased mortality from cardiovascular disease (twofold), respiratory disease (threefold) and infectious disease (fourfold). Therefore, as well as enhancing public mental health in order to improve population health and well-being, psychiatric services need to pay close attention to the physical health monitoring of patients.

Systems approach to improving safety

Tackling patient safety issues such as those detailed in this chapter requires the adoption of a systematic approach to analysing, assessing and mitigating patient safety risks in order to achieve reliable and safe care for patients. Many innovative healthcare organisations have made important breakthroughs in the design and performance of safer systems by focusing on lessons learned in other high-reliability industries with a long history of using quality improvement methodology. This has led to the introduction of initiatives such as standardising approaches, process re-engineering, decreasing complexity, incorporating human factors design and focusing on developing a safety culture. The 'seven steps' framework (Figure 19.3) aims to help healthcare organisations adopt a systems approach to improving patient safety.

Patient safety in primary care

Figure 20.1 Patient safety learning in general practice

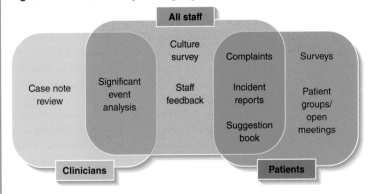

Box 20.1 Example of patient safety incident report from general practice

"Patient on oral methotrexate admitted to hospital diagnosed with Severe Community Acquired Pneumonia. Was prescribed Cefalexin 250 mg four times daily and Nystatin mouthwash for sore mouth, tongue, and throat pain by their GP surgery on morning of admission. Antibiotic/antifungal therapy was given following a telephone consultation. Patient not seen in person and there was no urgent Full Blood Count taken"

Figure 20.2 Example of drug interaction alert linked to electronic medical record

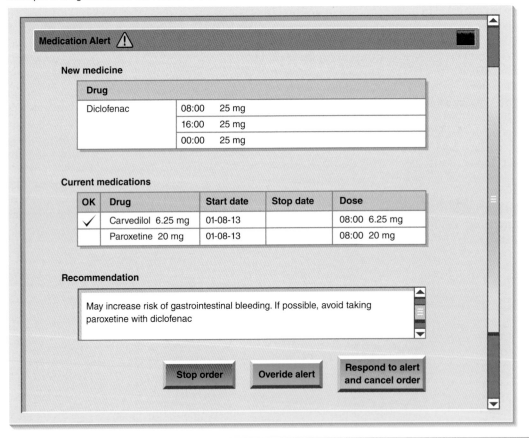

Patient Safety and Healthcare Improvement at a Glance, First Edition. Edited by Sukhmeet S. Panesar, Andrew Carson-Stevens, Sarah A. Salvilla and Aziz Sheikh
© 2014 John Wiley & Sons, Ltd. Published 2014 by John Wiley & Sons, Ltd.

Introduction

Around one in 50 patient encounters in primary care involve a patient safety incident, with substantial patient harm occurring for one in 20 of those incidents. With 303.9 million consultations occurring per year in general practices in England alone (2008–2009), approximately six million patients will experience a patient safety incident and around three hundred thousand are likely to result in substantial harm to patients. General practice consultations represent a subset of the encounters in primary care, so the actual burden from errors in this setting, including pharmacy, nursing, dentistry, out-of-hours services and community hospitals, for example, is likely to be substantially higher than the estimates suggests.

Factors influencing the risk of patient safety problems

General practice is the most common first level of contact with patients, and is unsurprisingly the largest specialty in most health-care systems. The way general practice is delivered can vary in terms of models of delivery (e.g. via general practice surgeries, community hospitals and GP-led health centres); the number of patients being served; the availability of services offered, and specialist services and secondary care support; the diversity of patients (e.g. ethnic groups and chronic disease profile); and the size and skill mix of the healthcare professional team providing care.

In recent years, there has been an emphasis on general practice teams providing and facilitating more complex care. This often involves coordinating input from primary, secondary and social care sectors. Additional issues include the variety of undifferentiated complaints that patients can present with, accepting diagnostic uncertainty, acting as the gatekeeper for further investigations, specialist opinion or emergency assessment and managing multiple comorbidities. As a result of these issues, the potential risk of patient safety problems occurring inevitably increases.

Building a safety culture in general practice

General practice delivery often involves teams of healthcare professionals (GPs, nurses, nursing assistants, community midwifes and psychologists), as well as others such as administrative staff, practice managers and office caretakers. The team's awareness of the potential for things to go wrong, and their ability to identify and acknowledge mistakes, learn from them and introduce changes to improve the situation next time, are essential to increasing patient safety.

A general practice team with a strong safety culture might demonstrate the following attributes:

• *Commitment*: Buy-in to the philosophy that safer, better quality care is possible, and improvement tools exist to deliver this vision for their patients.

• *Teamwork*: Everyone in the team – clinicians and non-clinicians – are clear on the contributions they can make to improving the quality of care delivery. This might include knowing that a staff suggestion box exists to improve work processes in-house, knowing how to access the incident reporting system via a practice computer and knowing who to discuss potential problems within the practice.

• *Leadership*: Each team member's personal commitment to patient safety is reflected in their preparedness to assume ownership when problems occur. Individual members might work to champion patient safety by ensuring it is a standing agenda item at all practice meetings, carrying out significant event audits that are led around priority issues identified by the wider team and having advocate training for all staff on methods to improve patient safety.

• *Accountability*: Taking responsibility for your actions at a professional, legal, ethical and contractual level. This might include: writing a patient safety incident report when an incident occurs; leading significant event audits in areas that could put patients at risk of harm; being open with patients when an error occurs, and recognising the importance of saying sorry; and responsibly reflecting on complaints made by patients and service users.

• *Understanding*: Recognising that 'every system is perfectly designed to achieve the results it gets'. This requires team members to look beyond blaming an individual and seek to identify the system factors that led to an event occurring. Individuals should recognise that when the workload is high, the risk of error increases, and work processes need to be flexible and adaptable to meet the demands of the service.

• *Communication*: Openness to share good practice and voice concerns or opportunities for improvement through recognised channels of communication. Patient safety should feature as a standing agenda item in practice meetings and feature in the annual practice report.

Methods for safer practice

There are several ways to improve patient safety in general practice, which can include:

• Make patient safety a standing agenda item at all practice meetings.

• Reflect on results from audits of medical records that seek to: identify avoidable acute admissions and preventable deaths (e.g. poly-pharmacy in elderly) or patients lost to follow up (e.g. patients on lithium or anti-coagulation therapy); and detect and measure harm (read more about the global trigger tool in Chapter 16).

• Discuss the learning from significant event audits and incident reports (see Box 20.1) at practice meetings and other meetings for local learning (with multiple other practices), and at a national level (e.g. the National Reporting and Learning System; read more about reporting systems in Chapter 6).

• Use technology to reduce risk to patients, such as computerised decision support tools to minimise risk of prescribing errors (read more about medical errors in Chapter 11; see Figure 20.2 for example interaction).

• Provide patients and all team members with ways to give their views on improving patient safety (e.g. patient safety, incident report forms and focus groups), and feedback the risks identified to them, the changes subsequently implemented and the lessons learned.

• Have a clear policy for providing a prompt, full, honest and compassionate explanation of any incidents, with an apology in a timely manner.

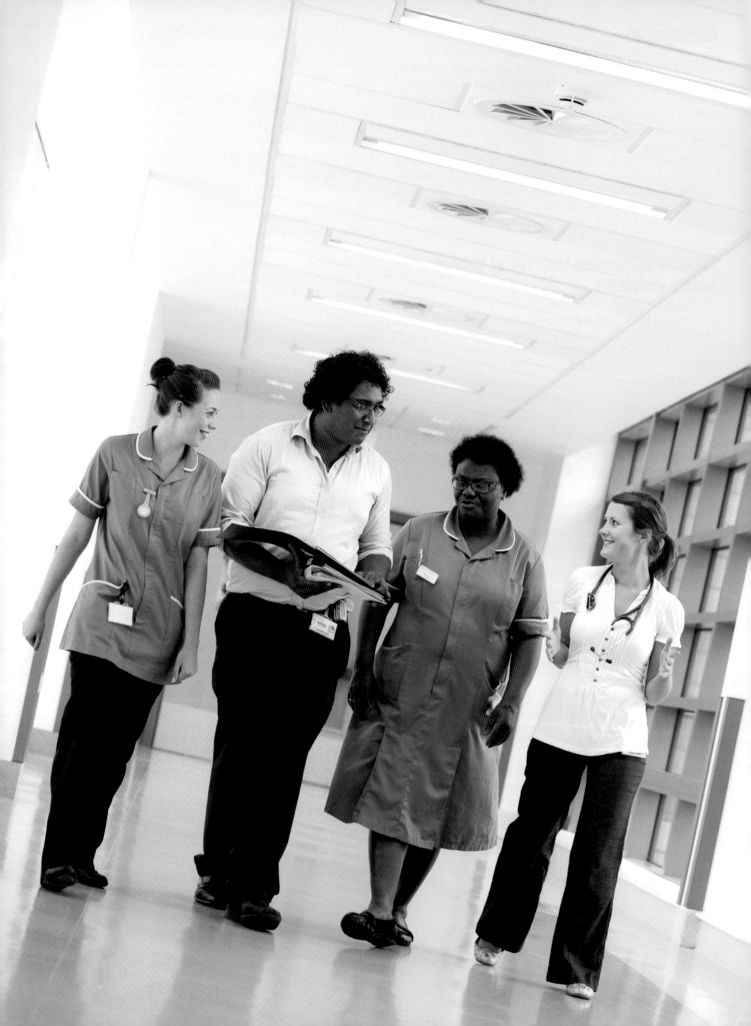

Quality improvement

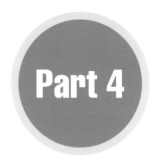
Part 4

Chapters

21 # Improving the quality of clinical care

Table 21.1 Aims of quality improvement: examples of what they mean to patients and healthcare professionals

Aim	Definition	Intervention	What this can mean for the patient and their family	What this means for the healthcare professional
Safe	To avoid unintentional harm from care provided to patients	Paediatric Early Warning Score (PEWS) *(See Chapter 16)*	A healthcare team member is regularly assessing the child	A patient showing early signs of deterioration receives escalated care and intervention
Patient and family centred	Providing care that is respectful of the needs and values of the patient and their family	Patient stories to identify opportunities to improve the care experience *(See Chapter 28)*	Opportunity to share experiences to improve the experience for future patients	Move from asking, 'What's the matter?' to 'What matters to you?'
Efficient	Avoiding waste	Process mapping in operating rooms *(See Chapter 36)*	Fewer cancelled operations and shorter waiting lists	More elective procedures per day and increased capacity for emergency cases
Effective	Providing care informed by the best available evidence which provides clear benefits	Central venous catheter care bundle *(See Chapters 18 and 34)*	Shorter overall hospital stay	The bundle is a reminder that simple tasks done reliably can decrease length of stay in ICU and overall hospital stay, and minimise risk of death
Timely	Reducing harmful delays	Cardiotocography (CTG) sticker *(See Chapters 13 and 35)*	Baby in distress is identified and delivered as soon as possible	The visual aid supports complex decision making in potentially stressful situations
Equity	Providing high-quality care regardless of a patient's characteristics	Suicide prevention strategies amongst mental health patients *(See Chapter 19)*	Support and care are provided in and out of hospital when assessed to be at risk of suicide	A coordinated, multidisciplinary action plan is initiated for those at high risk of suicide

Source: Adapted from the Institute of Medicine 2001 report, Crossing the Quality Chasm: A New Health System for the 21st Century.

Figure 21.1 A patient's journey through an improvement active hospital

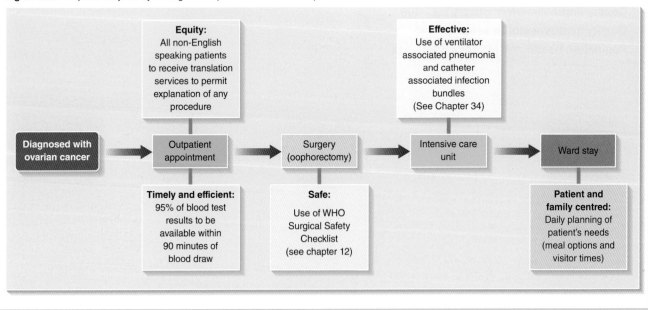

Patient Safety and Healthcare Improvement at a Glance, First Edition. Edited by Sukhmeet S. Panesar, Andrew Carson-Stevens, Sarah A. Salvilla and Aziz Sheikh
© 2014 John Wiley & Sons, Ltd. Published 2014 by John Wiley & Sons, Ltd.

Introduction

Despite the hard work, compassion and commitment of busy healthcare professionals, problems in the systems they train and work in often lead to a less than optimal experience for patients. The moral and ethical compass of those in the caring profession is shaped by the precept 'First, do no harm'. So it is not surprising that statistics such as '1 in 10 patients acutely admitted to hospital are harmed' alarm clinicians and expose a contradiction of the fundamental expectations of healthcare.

The focus on improving safety in healthcare has been invaluable. However, overall quality improvement in healthcare can be described through six aims (adapted from the Institute of Medicine; see Table 21.1). It is when patient care deviates from the six aims that healthcare professionals rightly become frustrated with an inability to 'do the right thing', and wonder what improvements could be made 'if only we could change things around here'. It's encouraging that many healthcare professionals no longer merely express frustration with the clearly evident problems they see in their systems. These professionals act. They understand that they have two jobs – their clinical job (i.e. working with patients to co-produce health) and their improvement job (i.e. working collaboratively to improve systems and processes so patient care and outcomes get better). So we now have a healthcare workforce that is increasingly aware of the responsibility, the duty, to improve. But knowing how to make improvements is not something most people are trained in. So how might you act to improve healthcare?

The science of improvement and the Model for Improvement

Everyone involved in the planning and delivery of healthcare must continuously seek ways to improve the systems within which they work. One proven approach to do this is the science of improvement. The science of improvement combines expert 'subject matter knowledge' (i.e. your insights and know-how of the clinical issue to be improved) with improvement methods and tools to create an approach that emphasises innovation, rapid-cycle testing in varying contexts and spread. The science of improvement is derived from W. Edwards Deming's system of profound knowledge which requires an understanding of systems, an understanding of variation, a theory of knowledge and an understanding of psychology ('profound knowledge' is discussed in more detail in Chapter 22).

Healthcare is complex, but using expert subject knowledge and the elements of Deming's 'profound knowledge' to build as complete a picture as possible of the problem you want to improve is logical. But once you have identified issues to improve on, it can be difficult to operationalise your intentions into actions. This is why many to most well-intentioned efforts result in either a lot of talk about change with no actual changes, or a lot of changes implemented but with very little actual improvement. One of the 'improvement methods and tools' at the heart of the science of improvement is the Model for Improvement, developed by Associates for Process Improvement ('disciples' of Deming's) and described in more detail in Chapter 23. Three questions form the core of the Model for Improvement:

1 What are we trying to accomplish?
2 How will we know that a change is an improvement?
3 What changes can we make that will result in improvement?

The other core element of the model is a series of plan–do–study–act (PDSA) cycles that inform the degree of belief that the changes proposed in Question 3 have the desired influence (increase or decrease) on the measures identified by Question 2, thus edging closer (or otherwise) towards achieving the project aim identified in Question 1. PDSA cycles are meant to be short and rapid, with each cycle producing knowledge that updates the 'theory of knowledge' and the design of the improvement effort.

Measurement techniques and statistical analysis will help you to determine which changes (and when) are leading to the improvements you seek (more detail in Chapter 24). There is a temptation to rush to generate a summary of the changes that led to improvements in order to spread the intervention to other settings. But the Model for Improvement emphasises the importance of always starting small in differing contexts in order to generate the necessary knowledge for those contexts (see Chapter 25).

Supporting your use of the Model for Improvement

There are many improvement tools to support your use of the Model for Improvement (e.g. to inform your answers to each question and design your PDSA cycles). A sample of tools is described in Chapters 26–32 to visualise, understand and assess the current system and plan changes. Patient stories have also proven to be a powerful method for accelerating improvement efforts by highlighting issues that would otherwise be overlooked by statistical methods (Chapter 28). Great societal leaders have demonstrated powerful methods of communicating urgency for change using stories. Those who are leading improvement projects should use stories to catalyse their improvement efforts (see Chapters 29 and 30).

Successful improvement projects are often run by a multidisciplinary team representative of those working within the system that is being changed (see Chapter 31 for tips on planning your project). The importance of engaging a multi-disciplinary team and giving every team member a role and a voice cannot be overstated. At the Institute for Healthcare Improvement, they call this essential approach 'all teach, all learn' – it is an acknowledgement that in improvement, everyone has something to teach, and everyone has something to learn.

Whilst planning is essential, managing lots of ideas and people, delivering the change as well as addressing barriers during the project can be challenging. Having a set of tools to visualise your theories for change (e.g. a driver diagram), as well as project management methods (e.g. a Gantt chart) to ensure you and your colleagues stay focused on the aim, can help keep track of your improvement progress (Chapter 32). Improving healthcare is hard work, and finding inspiration in the leadership efforts of others is crucial. Borrow ideas, share the learning as widely as you can (via conference presentations, journal articles, blogging etc.) and be sure to support other colleagues who are also interested in participating in, or leading, improvement (Chapters 33–37).

Figure 21.1 charts a patient's journey through an improvement active healthcare setting; whilst an improvement project might focus on one specific quality aim, many will reflect multiple aims.

22 Science of improvement

Figure 22.1 Lens of profound knowledge

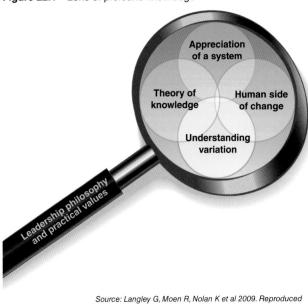

Source: Langley G, Moen R, Nolan K et al 2009. Reproduced with permission of John Wiley & Sons Ltd.

Figure 22.2 Subject matter knowledge, profound knowledge and improvement

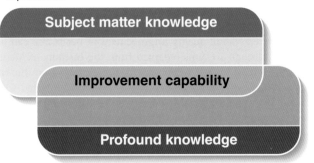

Figure 22.3 Adverse drugs events per 1000 patients

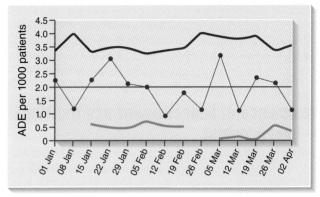

Figure 22.4 Special cause patterns

1. A single point outside the control limits

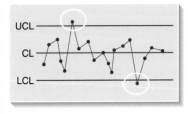

2. A run of eight or more points in a row above (or below) the centreline

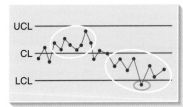

3. Six consecutive points increasing (trend up) or decreasing (trend down)

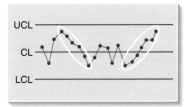

4. Two out of three consecutive points near (outer one-third) a control limit

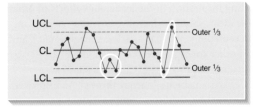

5. Fifteen consecutive points close (inner one-third of the chart) to the timeline

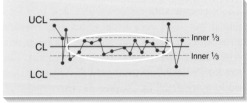

Source: Lloyd P. Provost and Sandra K. Murray (2011). The Health Care Data Guide: Learning from data for Improvement. Jossey-Bass. Reproduced with permission of John Wiley & Sons Ltd.

Patient Safety and Healthcare Improvement at a Glance, First Edition. Edited by Sukhmeet S. Panesar, Andrew Carson-Stevens, Sarah A. Salvilla and Aziz Sheikh
© 2014 John Wiley & Sons, Ltd. Published 2014 by John Wiley & Sons, Ltd.

Introduction

- To improve healthcare, there are four components of knowledge that a leader can use to guide change:
- Theory of variation
- Systems theory
- Theory of knowledge
- Psychology

Figure 22.1 shows how these four theories interact with each other. A leader's philosophy and practical values guide the use of this knowledge. W. Edwards Deming commented that we don't have to be experts in these fields:

> *One need not be eminent in any part of profound knowledge in order to understand it and to apply it. The various segments of the system of profound knowledge cannot be separated. They interact with each other. For example knowledge about psychology is incomplete without knowledge of variation.*

The system of profound knowledge provides a map to understanding and optimising organisations. When leading an improvement project, you should understand the basic theories in each area, how the different areas interrelate and why they are important for the improvement of quality.

Leaders combine subject matter knowledge and profound knowledge in creative ways to develop effective changes for improvement (see Figure 22.2). Subject matter knowledge is the knowledge basic to the things we do in life and daily work (e.g. how to drive a car, how to programme an infusion pump, understanding paediatric dosing regimes and scheduling outpatient appointments), and profound knowledge describes the intellectual depth and insight gained from understanding theories of systems, variation, knowledge and psychology.

Attributes of a leader with profound knowledge

Variation

Healthcare is dynamic and complex. Leaders understand that variation can help explain the changes seen in project measures because of *common causes* and *special causes*:

- **Common causes**: those causes that are inherent in the process over time, that affect everyone working in the process and that affect all outcomes of the process. Figure 22.3 shows a control chart that is dominated by common cause variation. It shows a chart that is in statistical control (a stable process) and is averaging two adverse drug events per 1000 patients
- **Special causes**: those causes that are *not* part of the process all the time or do not affect everyone, but arise because of specific circumstances. Figure 22.4 describes five possible patterns that would be identified as special causes (explained with further rules in more detail in Chapter 24)

Graphical methods help one to learn from data and can be used by others to consider variation in their decisions and actions. Leaders understand the concept of stable and unstable processes, and the potential losses due to tampering. When stakes from making changes are high, advanced methods can be used to measure the capability of a process or system before changes are attempted.

Systems

Leaders study and manage their organisation as a system. They emphasise the importance of common purpose and interdependencies among groups in the organisation. They understand that the performance of the organisation depends more on the interaction of the various parts than how the parts perform individually. They understand both detail and dynamic complexity in a system. They consider important systems concepts such as boundaries, feedback loops, constraints and leverage points, and use these concepts to develop, test and implement changes to optimise the system. Figure 22.5 shows the shift in focus from describing the organisation in a hierarchical organisation chart to the organisation being viewed as a system that is focused on patients.

Knowledge

Leaders understand that management is prediction that comes from knowledge, and knowledge is built on theory. They understand that people learn in different ways. They use the plan–do–study–act (PDSA) cycle for learning and improvement to learn, run tests on a small scale and make decisions (described in more detail in Chapter 23). In order to enhance learning, they make predictions before changes are made. Figure 22.6 shows the iterative nature of learning and how deductive and inductive learning are built into the PDSA cycle.

The leader understands that organisational learning depends on a shared understanding of key terms used. Operational definitions are necessary to create shared meaning. An operational definition should include:

- A method of measurement or test
- A set of criteria for judgement

For example, what do we mean by a 'patient fall'? This seems simple enough. Consider the following definitions of a fall:

- "….a sudden uncontrolled, unintentional downward displacement of the body to the ground or other object, excluding falls resulting from violent blows or other purposeful actions"
- "….inadvertently coming to rest on the ground, floor or other lower level, excluding intentional change in position to rest in furniture, wall or other objects"

How a fall is defined can be very different from the perspective of the patient or caregivers. The elderly may consider a fall to be the

Figure 22.5   Change of organisational view to a systems view focused on patients

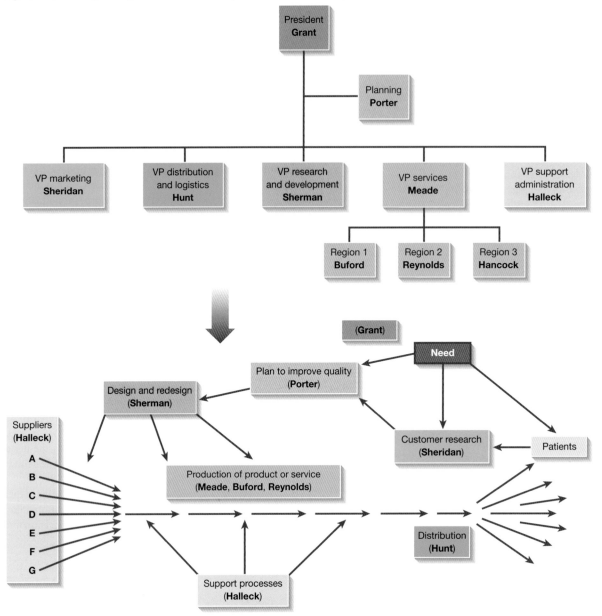

Source: Maccoby M, Norman CL, Norman CJ & Margolies R 2013. Reproduced with permission of John Wiley & Sons Ltd.

Figure 22.6   Plan–do–study–act (PDSA), deductive and inductive learning

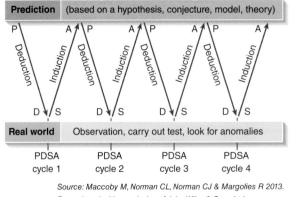

Source: Maccoby M, Norman CL, Norman CJ & Margolies R 2013.
Reproduced with permission of John Wiley & Sons Ltd.

'loss of balance'. If you are interpreting data from your organisation on falls, then the definition becomes important. Have we created a definition that is focused on patients? Have the definition and the measure masked our safety relative to falls? Has the definition caused an overreaction resulting in wasted time by healthcare professionals?

How we learn with deductive and inductive learning theory, and the use of operational definitions, only scratches the surface of the ideas that could be placed under the description of 'theory of knowledge'. There is much more to learn, so this is a start.

Psychology

Leaders appreciate how to create an environment that is conducive to unleashing the power of intrinsic motivation. Michael Maccoby has described the 'Five Rs of Motivation' for leaders:

1 Reasons: People are motivated to support change when the reasons for that change make sense to them.

2 Responsibilities: People want to know how change will affect their responsibilities

3 Relationships: People are motivated by good relationships with supervisors, collaborators and the people they serve.

4 Recognition: People enjoy having their contributions to the system recognised. Recognition enhances the dignity of the individual, one of the basic human drives.

5 Rewards: It is essential that people consider all pay and rewards to be fair. Giving out bonuses can strengthen a supervisor's authority, but it won't motivate workers to do their work any better. Worse, they may be demotivated by the pressure to conform to a job that is not intrinsically motivating.

Leaders also have what Maccoby has called 'personality intelligence'. Personality intelligence is essential for creating motivation. Personality intelligence includes both concepts and emotional understanding, both head and heart. The concepts include:

• **Talents and temperament** – what we are born with
• **Social character** – how we are like others brought up in the same culture
• **Drives** – how we are like all people
• **Motivational type** – how we are like some people within our culture
• **Identity and philosophy** – how we are no one else

Summary

Four parts of profound knowledge have been discussed:

• Theory of variation – special versus common cause variation
• Systems theory – viewing the organisation as a system
• Theory of knowledge – appreciating the way in which the PDSA cycle builds theory for effective action
• Psychology – the important role of motivation and personality intelligence in working with people; probably 80% of the effort in making effective changes

23 Model for Improvement

Figure 23.1 Model for Improvement

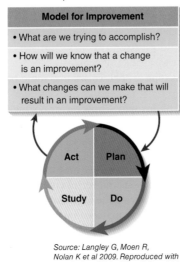

Source: Langley G, Moen R, Nolan K et al 2009. Reproduced with permission of John Wiley & Sons Ltd.

Figure 23.2 Definition of improvement

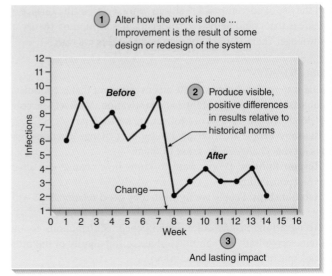

Source: Langley G, Moen R, Nolan K et al 2009. Reproduced with permission of John Wiley & Sons Ltd.

Table 23.1 How will we know a change is an improvement?

Goals	Measures	Type of measure
Decrease CAUTI rate	• Time between CAUTI rate	Outcome
Decrease inappropriate catheter use	• Catheter days/100 patient days	Process
Increase nurses' knowledge on criteria for catheter use	• Score of the pre and post test	Process
Increase nurses' compliance to new process on review of catheter use	• % nurse compliant to new process on review of catheter	Process
Maintain or increase staff satisfaction	• Nurse satisfaction score • Physician satisfaction score	Balancing

Figure 23.3 The plan–do–study–act cycle

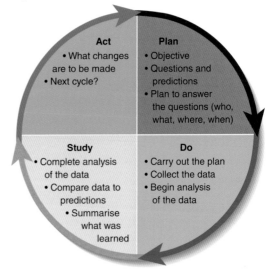

Source: Langley G, Moen R, Nolan K et al 2009. Reproduced with permission of John Wiley & Sons Ltd.

Patient Safety and Healthcare Improvement at a Glance, First Edition. Edited by Sukhmeet S. Panesar, Andrew Carson-Stevens, Sarah A. Salvilla and Aziz Sheikh
© 2014 John Wiley & Sons, Ltd. Published 2014 by John Wiley & Sons, Ltd.

Introduction

All improvement requires change, and change can involve the design or redesign of a process. However, you need to be confident that the changes you are making will lead to the improvement you seek. You need to consider:

* Why these changes?
* How will we know the changes presented have improved patient care?

By asking these questions routinely whenever making changes or applying new knowledge, learning can be generated about what really helped to deliver results.

The Model for Improvement (Figure 23.1) is a method used worldwide in healthcare when making changes that affect patients. It has three fundamental questions which will help focus on what exactly the change is seeking to improve. The three questions may involve a series of plan–do–study–act (PDSA) cycles, where you develop, test and implement changes. It is rare to be able to answer the three questions without running PDSA cycles – few projects are that simple. Figure 23.2 defines what the improvement is following the change.

1. What are we trying to accomplish?

The answer to the question must state what process, product, service or system will be designed or redesigned. Table 23.2 describes some useful and less useful responses to this question.

Table 23.2 What are we trying to accomplish?

Less Useful Response for Question 1	Better Response for Question 1
Reduce infections	Redesign the existing urinary catheter review and removal of criteria to reduce CAUTI in surgical recovery wards.

2. How will we know that a change is an improvement?

When answering this question, there are three levels of measurement to consider: **outcome measures** relate directly to the aim of the improvement effort, **process measures** determine whether activities have been accomplished as planned and **balancing measures** ensure that changes are acceptable to those who must make the changes and ensures that changes do not cause unintended consequences. Table 23.2 provides examples of goals and measures that relate to reducing catheter-associated urinary tract infections.

3. What changes can we make that will result in improvement?

To answer this question, new changes must be developed that can then be tested, or known changes that are successfully being used by others can be tested. For relatively simple systems, a list of changes may be developed and tested almost immediately. Table 23.3 identifies changes that were tested to reduce catheter-associated urinary tract infections.

The plan–do–study–act cycle

Once the three fundamental questions are answered, the PDSA cycle (Figure 23.3) is then the primary means for turning ideas into action and connecting action to learning. The PDSA cycle simplifies the scientific method to test ideas and determine what action should be taken. Using the cycle effectively takes some discipline and effort. The PDSA form in Figure 23.4 provides some detail on what should be considered in each phase of the cycle.

Table 23.3 Changes to test (PDSAs)

Test new urinary catheter decision-making algorithm
To test effectiveness of training on improving nurses' knowledge of appropriate indication on urinary catheter use
Test integrating the results of the nurses' daily catheter review into doctor-led ward rounds
Test installing a computer screen reminder

The purpose of each cycle is to build your degree of belief that changes you are making are leading to the improvements you predicted. This will allow you to identify which changes were effective and reject those that failed to meet predictions. In Chapter 25, you will consider why this is important as you spread changes to other clinical settings, hospitals and even other countries.

Figure 23.4 PDSA form

Cycle #1 Objective: Test new urinary catheter decision-making algorithm

PLAN

Learning Questions:

1. How will this change reduce catheter utilisation and CAUTI? Why?
Prediction: Nurses currently wait for doctors to identify when a catheter should be removed. We think this will reduce utilisation from 1–2 days less. The longer catheters are in, the more likely CAUTIs can occur.

2. How will this change increase nurses' knowledge on criteria of urinary catheter removal? Why?
Currently, doctors are solely responsible for determining when a catheter is removed. A catheter removal algorithm will guide the nurses.

3. How will this change increase nurses' compliance to the new process on review of catheter use? Why?
Nurses will help develop a catheter review form to be used by nurses and use it to test with all the nurses. Because they helped develop it, they will own it.

4. How will this change impact doctor and nurse satisfaction? Why?
Doctors will like this since they will not be solely responsible for determining time to remove, & nurses will like this since they will be able to remove the catheter earlier.

Test Plan:
1. The algorithm that is being used in other locations will be reviewed by the Medical Director and Nurse Sponsor and altered to match the conditions.
2. A new review form will be developed to make it easy for the nurses to follow the algorithm.
3. The Medical Director and Nurse Sponsor will approve the review form. And pre-test it with one nurse and her patients on Day x.
4. All nurses on day shift will be tested for their knowledge, then trained (with a post-test) to understand the decision-making criteria and how to use the form, by a senior nurse supervisor. Doctors will be informed about the change on Day y.
5. Test will be conducted for Day z. Results will be reviewed, and the test will be extended if it is successful.

Data Collection Plan:
Nurse knowledge (pre & post training); catheter utilisation rate (pre-post test); time between CAUTIs; new process compliance (for extended test); staff satisfaction.

DO: (Execute the Plan)
Observations/Surprises: Doctors who asked nurses for their catheter review results caused those nurses to be more confident and open. After the first day, the nurses asked to extend the test to more patients.

(continued)

STUDY: (what was learned?)

Learning questions:

1. No CAUTIs have been reported. On the first day, 5 catheters were removed from patients

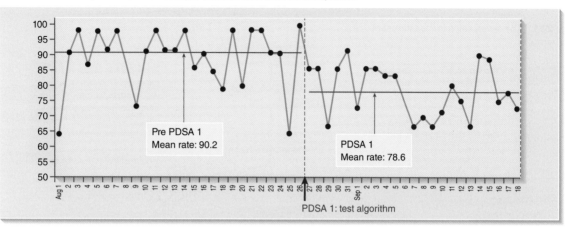

Pre PDSA 1
Mean rate: 90.2

PDSA 1
Mean rate: 78.6

PDSA 1: test algorithm

2. Nurse scores have increased

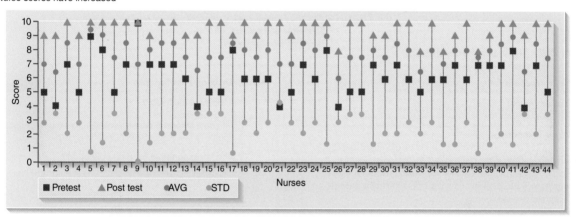

Score

■ Pretest ▲ Post test ● AVG ● STD

Nurses

3. Percentage of inappropriate indication with corrective action taken (compliance)

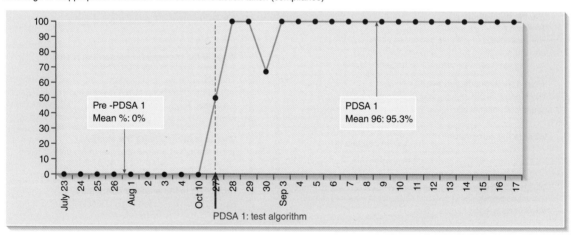

Pre -PDSA 1
Mean %: 0%

PDSA 1
Mean 96: 95.3%

PDSA 1: test algorithm

4. Doctors are positive and want to move catheter review to ward rounds. Nurses want to implement the new protocol

ACT:

1. Test adding the catheter review results in daily ward rounds for doctors to continue to build confidence in nurses

2. Test adding an electronic reminder on the handover system to remind the team to conduct a catheter review

24 Measurement for improvement

Figure 24.1 The seven steps to measurement

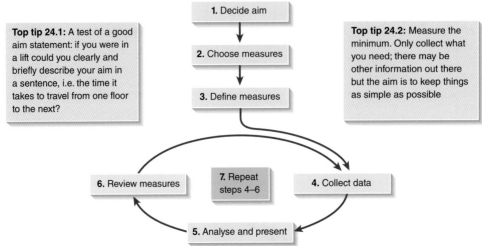

Top tip 24.1: A test of a good aim statement: if you were in a lift could you clearly and briefly describe your aim in a sentence, i.e. the time it takes to travel from one floor to the next?

Top tip 24.2: Measure the minimum. Only collect what you need; there may be other information out there but the aim is to keep things as simple as possible

1. Decide aim

2. Choose measures

3. Define measures

6. Review measures

7. Repeat steps 4–6

4. Collect data

5. Analyse and present

Figure 24.2 The measures checklist

Part 1: Measure setup	Part 2: Measurement process
Measure name: DNA rate for clinic A	**Is the data available?** *(currently available/available with minor changes/prospective collection needed)* Both data items are readily available from the outpatient module of the Patient Administration System
Why is it important? We need to ensure that the clinic is not disrupted by having unexpected gaps in the clinic schedule. The policy for this clinic is to offer another appointment which means that other patients may be disadvantaged if we have too many patients being rescheduled	**Who is responsible for data collection?** The Information Analyst attached to the project team
Who owns this measure? The outpatient manager	**What is the process of collection?** The analyst will extract the relevant data weekly using existing reporting sofware
What is the definition? *(spell it out very clearly in words)* The percentage of patients booked to attend clinic A who did not attend for their appointment and no warning was received at the clinic before it started	**What is the process for presenting results?** *(e.g. create run chart or bar chart in Excel)* The DNA rate will be plotted on a run chart with each point representing the actual DNA rate for each clinic. The clinic runs twice a week so there will be two data points plotted per week
What data items do you need? The number of patients booked to attend clinic (B) and the number of patients who failed to attend without warning (F)	**Who is responsible for the analysis?** The Information Analyst attached to the project team
What is the calculation? $$\frac{100 \times \text{DNA patients (F)}}{\text{Booked patients (B)}}$$	**How often is the analysis completed?** New data will be added every 2 weeks
Which patient groups are to be covered? Do you need to stratify? *(e.g. are there differences by shift, time of day, day of week, severity, etc)* All patients booked into the clinic	**Where will decisions be made based on results?** The project team meets every fortnight and the data is a standing item on the agenda
What is the numeric goal you are setting yourselves? We want to achieve no more than 5% DNAs	**Who is responsible for taking action?** The project team leader together with the outpatient clinic manager
Who is responsible for setting this? The Outpatient Improvement project team	
When will it be achieved by? Within 9 months from the start of the project	

Left margin labels: Measure definition / Goal setting
Right margin labels: Collect / Analyse – Calculate measure and present results / Review

Patient Safety and Healthcare Improvement at a Glance, First Edition. Edited by Sukhmeet S. Panesar, Andrew Carson-Stevens, Sarah A. Salvilla and Aziz Sheikh
© 2014 John Wiley & Sons, Ltd. Published 2014 by John Wiley & Sons, Ltd.

Introduction

Measurement is a fundamental component of the Model for Improvement, by answering the question 'How do we know that a change is an improvement?' To answer this, it is useful to collect and use the right data, but good data do not happen by chance – they are the result of a sound process. Using a process called the 'seven steps to measurement' (Figure 24.1) should help you to collect data that are good enough to use for your improvement project. A measures checklist also accompanies the seven steps model (Figure 24.2).

Steps 1 to 3 – Getting ready

Step 1 – Decide your aim

This is a direct reference to the first question in the Model for Improvement. Unless you are very clear what you are setting out to achieve, then you are unlikely to be able to decide what to measure. Create an aim statement that is unambiguous, specific, succinct and measurable. Not sure how good your aim statement is? Try the exercise in Top Tip 24.1.

Step 2 – Choose your measures

Your aim will probably have suggested an obvious measure or measures. However, there are other tools to help you:
• Chapter 32 introduces the **driver diagram**. If you have created one of these, you can use it to identify likely measures. Measures attached to drivers will mostly be outcome measures, and those attached to interventions will be process measures
• If you have undertaken a **process-mapping** exercise (see Chapter 26) as part of your improvement work, this can also be useful in suggesting possible measures

You need to ensure a balance between outcome and process measures. Think you've not got enough measures? Check out Top Tip 24.2.

Step 3 – Define your measures

This is an area that can cause problems, particularly when using a common measure such as 'length of stay' because there are many definitions that might be used. Will the length of stay in hospital or in a particular ward be included, and will it be measured in whole days or in hours?

Measures always require common agreement on definitions. This means specifying exactly what is meant and applying this definition consistently. Make sure that your measure is well-defined and has clear instructions that can be easily followed and repeated both by yourself at a later date and by others.
• *Repeatability*: Can you, the person who created the definition, collect the right data consistently using it?
• *Reproducibility*: Can the definition that you have created be reproduced by other individuals?

Figure 24.2 shows the checklist completed for an improvement project undertaken in an outpatient department. The project team wanted to reduce the number of patients who did not attend (DNA) their appointments and have chosen the DNA rate as one of their project measures. In part 1 of the checklist, they have set out their rationale for choosing this measure and also defined it quite precisely. They have set themselves a goal, but they will not regard it as the only measure of success for their project. They know that they will learn a lot about why patients do not attend and that will help them design a process that works for patients.

Note that as well as defining the measure clearly, they have specified the data items required and also the calculation they will use to arrive at the DNA rate.

Sampling

When should we collect data on 100% of patients, and when should we use a sample? If your numbers are small enough or the data are easy enough to collect that you can cover 100% of patients, then you should do it. If this is not feasible, then you should use a sample. There is a lot written about how to select samples (see the 'Further reading' suggestions for this chapter at the end of the book), but essentially it is advisable to choose a sample that is representative of the overall population that you are measuring. This is so that you do not inadvertently introduce a bias into your results.

For example, you decide to choose five patients 'at random' from an outpatient clinic and take the top five case notes from the pile by reception. What you may not know is that the notes were placed in a particular order and you have chosen five female patients in a mixed-gender clinic. Does this matter? In some circumstances, it will. So use your judgement based on your knowledge of the process (i.e. your subject matter knowledge) you are sampling from.

One way you can avoid bias is to use a random number generator in spreadsheet software packages.

Steps 4 to 7 – The collect–analyse–review (CAR) measurement cycle

Measurement itself is a process. In its simplest form, it consists of three stages. First you collect the data, then you analyse them and present them in an appropriate way to convert them into useful information, and finally you review your information to see what decisions you need to make. The CAR cycle then starts all over again. The CAR cycle will help you to be explicit in your 'plan' about the data you need and how you 'do' collect and display it (Steps 4 and 5) to answer the questions and predictions you intend to review (Step 6) in order to 'study' and 'act' accordingly.

Step 4 – Collect your data

Once you have decided what data you need, you are all set to start collecting them. However, unless you already have a system set up to give you exactly the data you need, you will need to plan how to collect them. And that plan will need to answer the following questions:
• What are we collecting: data for every patient or just a sample?
• Who is actually going to get the data?
• How are they going to do it?
• Where will they get it from: historically stored in a database or collected in real time?

Test your plan, using plan–do–study–act (PDSA) principles, to ensure the data you get back are reliable and what you were expecting. Worried that collecting data is a burden? See Top Tip 24.3.

A word about baselines

You will need to know your baseline (i.e. how your process is currently performing) before you can track the progress toward your goal. To create a baseline, about 20–25 data points are ideal. This is because you want to see not just how you are doing 'on average', but also how variable your performance is and whether there are any cyclical trends to be aware of.

The number of points you need to demonstrate a difference will also depend on the size of the effect you expect to have (see Figure 24.4). Table 24.2 also gives further guidance on this

Table 24.1 Tests for number of runs above and below the median

Number of data points	Lower limit for number of runs	Upper limit for number of runs
10	3	8
11	3	9
12	3	10
13	4	10
14	4	11
15	4	12
16	5	12
17	5	13
18	6	13
19	6	14
20	6	15
21	7	15
22	7	16
23	8	16
24	8	17
25	9	17
26	9	18
27	9	19
28	10	19
29	10	20
30	11	20
31	11	21
32	11	22
33	11	22
34	12	23
35	13	23
36	13	24
37	13	25
38	14	25
39	14	26
40	15	26
41	16	26
42	16	27
43	17	27
44	17	28
45	17	29
46	17	30
47	18	30
48	18	31
49	19	31
50	19	32
60	24	37
70	28	43
80	33	46
90	37	54
100	42	59

Source: Perla RJ et al 2013. Qual Manag Health Care.

Top tip 24.3: Aim to make measurement part of the daily routine. Where possible, use mechanisms that are already in place or amend them. This minimises the burden on staff and also maximises the chances of it being done reliably

Top tip 24.4: Remember the goal is improvement and not a new measurement system. It's easy to get side-tracked into improving data quality, especially if you are confronted with challenges on the credibility of the data – just ensure it is 'good enough'

Figure 24.3 The number of complaints as a run chart

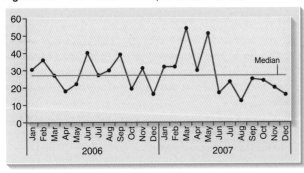

Figure 24.4 Attendances at an accident and emergency (A&E) department as a statistical process control (SPC) chart

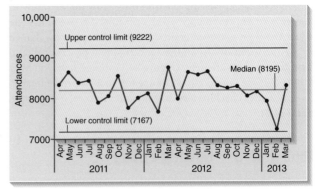

Table 24.2 Guidelines for number of data points to test a change (*Source: Adapted from Langley G, Moen R, Nolan K et al 2009. Reproduced with permission of John Wiley & Sons Ltd.*)

Total number of points	Situation
Fewer than ten	Expensive tests, expesive protoypes, or long time periods between available data points. Large effects anticpated.
Fifteen to fifty	Usually sufficient to discem patterns indicating improvements that are moderate or large.
Fifty to one hundred	The effect of the charge is expected to be small relative to the variation in the system.

Figure 24.5 Calculating moving ranges

Month	Jan	Feb	Mar	Apr	May	Jun	Jul
Value	31	36	27	18	22	40	27
Moving range		5	9	9	4	18	13

$$36 - 31 = +5 \qquad 27 - 36 = -9$$

Figure 24.6 Formulae for upper and lower control limits

$$\text{Upper control limit} = \text{Mean} + \frac{3 \times \text{Av MR}}{1.128}$$

$$\text{Lower control limit} = \text{Mean} - \frac{3 \times \text{Av MR}}{1.128}$$

based on the availability of data given the circumstances. One way to get more points is to measure more frequently.

Sometimes the data you need are not currently being collected. If so, you should start collecting your data straightaway. You can still start testing small changes. They will not affect your overall situation, so you can pursue those whilst creating your baseline.

Final word: do not go overboard on data collection. See Top Tip 24.4.

Step 5 – Analyse and present your data

Special-cause and common-cause variation (described in Chapter 22) are concepts used to distinguish between whether we have made a difference (special cause) or if the changes observed in our data are simply a result of random variation (common cause). Both run charts and statistical process control (SPC) charts can help to distinguish between these two types of variation.

Data are plotted in time order, and the median is represented as a straight line. Figure 24.3 provides an example of a run chart illustrating the number of complaints received each month in an organisation.

There are four statistical rules to identify possible special causes:

Test #1: Six or more consecutive points above or below the median. This indicates a shift in the process. Values are still varying, but they are doing so around a new median value. If this is a shift in the right direction, it is likely that the change you made is having a beneficial effect. This is the most frequent 'rule' that you will see after introducing a change.

Test #2: Five or more consecutive points all increasing or decreasing. This indicates a trend and suggests that the change you made is having an effect, but you don't know yet when performance will become stable again. You need to keep measuring to find out. This situation is more likely to occur if you are rolling out a change over a period of time.

Test #3: Too many or too few runs. A 'run' is a number of consecutive points on one side of the median. When counting, ignore any points that lie directly on the median. Use Table 24.1 to work out whether your variation is due to random causes. If the number of runs is inside the range, this is what we might expect by chance. If the number falls outside the range, then some external factor is having an effect. Too many runs suggest that the process has become less consistent, and it is possible that your change has had a detrimental effect. Too few runs suggest a more consistent process.

Test #4: An 'astronomical' data point. You use your own judgement to assess whether the data value in question really is 'odd'. Often, such markedly out-of-range results are caused by a data collection or data definition problem, so check that first. If the data seem ok then try to find out what might have caused such an odd result. It may cause you to think about creating a contingency plan for if such an occasion arose again.

Are any of these four rules present in the example given in Figure 24.3? Which months, if any, would you want to ask more questions about if these were data about a service you knew? Model answers are provided at the end of the chapter.

Statistical process control charts

Run charts should be sufficient for nearly all your measurement, but there may be occasion for you to need to understand how much variation the process of interest typically exhibits. For this, you will use an SPC chart. This chart (Figure 24.4) introduces the idea of expected variation. SPC charts still have a 'typical value' line (usually, the mean) but add two further lines, the upper and lower limits.

In Figure 24.4, we have plotted the monthly number of attendances at an accident and emergency (A&E) department over 2 years. The average number per month is 8195 attendances. The upper and lower limits show that attendances could vary by up to 1000 attendances on either side of the mean.

The purpose of these control limits is to show you that data points appearing within the limits, despite going up and down, are doing so as part of the normal variation that we see in everyday life. If a data point spikes above or below these limits, then you know something different has happened – a special event, hence this is called 'special-cause variation'. When events like this are seen on a chart, you need to investigate what happened. Even though the event might be unlikely to occur again, it is still worth considering if there is anything you can do to minimise the impact if it did.

If our process exhibits just random variation, we can use the SPC chart to 'predict' what future performance would be like. We would expect any future data points to vary around the average and lie within the limits.

Calculating the upper and lower limits

The upper and lower limits are derived from the actual data themselves. The more variable the data, the further apart the limits will be. There are several different types of SPC chart, each with its own way of calculating the limits and each designed for a specific type of data. However, there is one chart, called the XmR chart, that statistical process control experts like Don Wheeler suggest works for almost any type of data.

To calculate the upper and lower limits for this chart, do the following:

• Calculate the moving range for each pair of points in your data (see Figure 24.5)
• Calculate the average of the moving ranges ('Av MR' in Figure 24.6)
• Divide the Av MR by the bias correction constant, 1.128. Whatever your data, this is *always* the same value. This gives you one measure of variation (V)
• Add three measures of variation (3V) to the mean to get the upper limit, and subtract three measures of variation (3V) from the mean to get the lower limit. The formulae are shown in Figure 24.6

Special-cause rules

There are several statistical rules to identify possible special causes when using SPC charts. The eight rules described by Lloyd Nelson will help you to do this. The first three rules can be used without needing specialist SPC software and so are the most commonly used. Note that rules 1–3, 5 and 7 have already been illustrated in Chapter 22, but we include them here for completeness and convenience:

Rule #1: (Figure 24.7) – For any point outside one of the control limits, similar to an 'astronomical point' in run charts, SPC allows a statistical interpretation rather than just personal judgement.

Rule #2: (Figure 24.8) – A run of eight consecutive points all above or all below the centre line. This is the same as rule #1 for run charts and indicates a shift in the process. The actual number of points you take as a 'signal' (typically seven, eight or nine points are used) depends on your attitude towards risk. The more points you want to see, the less likely that sequence would happen by chance. For example, seven in a row occurs less than one in 100 times by chance.

Figure 24.7 Rule #1

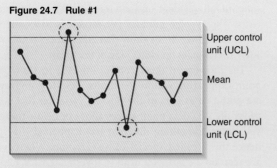

Upper control unit (UCL)

Mean

Lower control unit (LCL)

Figure 24.8 Rule #2

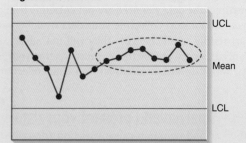

UCL

Mean

LCL

Figure 24.9 Rule #3

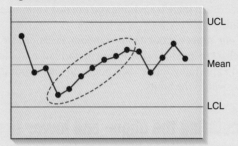

UCL

Mean

LCL

Figure 24.10 Rule #4

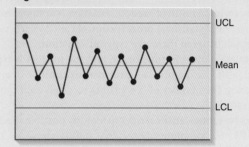

UCL

Mean

LCL

Figure 24.11 Showing measures of variation

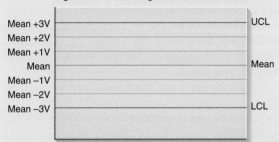

Mean +3V
Mean +2V
Mean +1V
Mean
Mean −1V
Mean −2V
Mean −3V

UCL

Mean

LCL

Figure 24.12 Rule #5

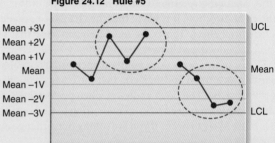

Mean +3V
Mean +2V
Mean +1V
Mean
Mean −1V
Mean −2V
Mean −3V

UCL

Mean

LCL

Figure 24.13 Rule #6

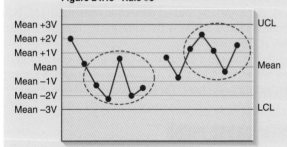

Mean +3V
Mean +2V
Mean +1V
Mean
Mean −1V
Mean −2V
Mean −3V

UCL

Mean

LCL

Figure 24.14 Rule #7

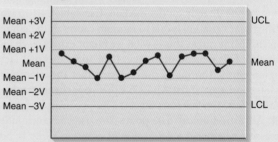

Mean +3V
Mean +2V
Mean +1V
Mean
Mean −1V
Mean −2V
Mean −3V

UCL

Mean

LCL

Figure 24.15 Rule #8

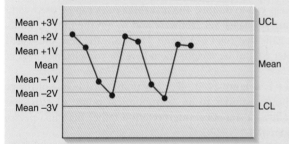

Mean +3V
Mean +2V
Mean +1V
Mean
Mean −1V
Mean −2V
Mean −3V

UCL

Mean

LCL

Rule #3: (Figure 24.9) – Six or more consecutive points all increasing or decreasing. This indicates a trend and is similar to rule #2 for run charts.

Rule #4: (Figure 24.10) – Fourteen points in a row alternating up and down. This is the classic sawtooth pattern that we often draw when sketching random variation freehand. In fact, this pattern is anything but random.

The following four rules now divide the space between the centre line (the average) and the control limits into three equal parts using the measure of variation calculated earlier (V). See Figure 24.11.

Rule #5: (Figure 24.12) – Two out of three consecutive points more than two measures of variation on the same side of the centre line. The size of the change means that it can be identified more quickly than rule #2.

Rule #6: (Figure 24.13) – Four out of five consecutive points more than one measure of variation on the same side of the centre line. The size of the change, although not as great as for rule #5, means that it can be identified more quickly than rule #2.

Rule #7: (Figure 24.14) – Fifteen consecutive points close to the centre line that are within one measure of variation. These points can be above or below the centre line. This happens when your process becomes more consistent or reliable.

Rule #8: (Figure 24.15) – Eight points in a row either above or below the centre line with *none* within one measure of variation. This indicates that the process has split in some way if it is a new phenomenon or that the data come from two sources, perhaps a morning shift and an afternoon shift, if it is present from the start. The solution in this case would be to plot the two shifts separately.

Step 6 – Review your data

It is vital that you set aside time to look at what your measures are telling you about your process and any impact changes that your processes may (or may not) have made. Remember that the purpose of measurement is to guide you to make the right decisions about your improvement project.

Step 7 – Keep going!

Repeat steps 4, 5 and 6 each month or more frequently. If you are measuring compliance with a process (e.g. compliance with handwashing or a care bundle), aim for a minimum of 95% for non-catastrophic processes. For a process where, if it fails, it will almost certainly result in serious injury or death, aim for 100%. Keep making changes until your data tell you this is so.

For outcomes (e.g. the surgical site infection rate or number of central line infections), you are aiming to consistently meet or exceed your goal. If you are using SPC charts, ensure the goal sits outside the appropriate upper or lower limit.

When do I stop measuring?

The simple answer is you don't. If you are consistently meeting your goal, you should still look to see if there are further improvements that could be made or monitor that things do not get worse again. Where you have a consistent performance in process measures, you may decide to measure less frequently. This is fine as long as there is a related outcome measure that you are continuing to monitor. If this shows signs of deteriorating, you may need to revisit the process measures.

Some measures that you choose will specifically relate to a change proposed within the project. For instance, you might be introducing a new piece of equipment and staff will need conversion training. Whilst you are running a series of PDSAs to learn about your efforts to convert staff, you might record data about compliance to key steps for safely using the new equipment. These would be 'PDSA-level measures' (as opposed to 'project-level measures'), and once you are satisfied that all staff are successfully trained, you do not need to continue measuring your progress.

Did you correctly interpret Figure 24.3?
There is a run of seven points below the median at the end of 2007. This is rule #1. There are 2 months (March and May 2007) that could be considered 'astronomical'. There are no special causes present before March 2007. You would want to be asking whether anything unusual was happening in March and May 2007 and did the organisation take any measures to improve services in May/June 2007?

25 Spread and sustainability of improvement

Figure 25.1 Ideas and their results in various settings

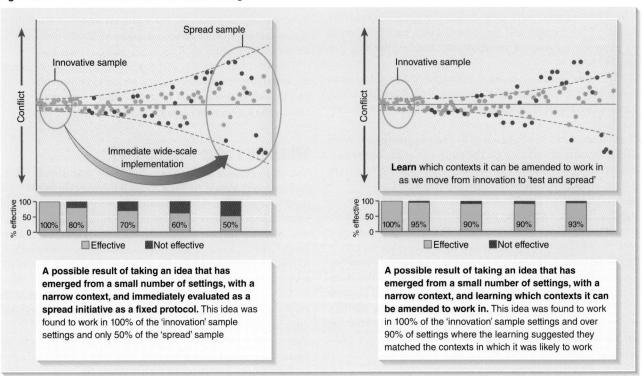

A possible result of taking an idea that has emerged from a small number of settings, with a narrow context, and immediately evaluated as a spread initiative as a fixed protocol. This idea was found to work in 100% of the 'innovation' sample settings and only 50% of the 'spread' sample

A possible result of taking an idea that has emerged from a small number of settings, with a narrow context, and learning which contexts it can be amended to work in. This idea was found to work in 100% of the 'innovation' sample settings and over 90% of settings where the learning suggested they matched the contexts in which it was likely to work

Source: Adapted from Parry GJ, Carson-Stevens A, Luff DF, et al (2013). Reproduced with permission of Elsevier.

Figure 25.2 Improvement phase by setting

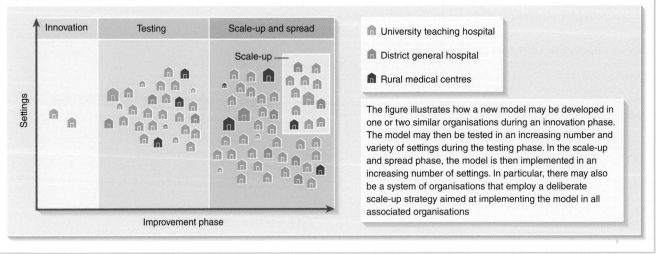

The figure illustrates how a new model may be developed in one or two similar organisations during an innovation phase. The model may then be tested in an increasing number and variety of settings during the testing phase. In the scale-up and spread phase, the model is then implemented in an increasing number of settings. In particular, there may also be a system of organisations that employ a deliberate scale-up strategy aimed at implementing the model in all associated organisations

Patient Safety and Healthcare Improvement at a Glance, First Edition. Edited by Sukhmeet S. Panesar, Andrew Carson-Stevens, Sarah A. Salvilla and Aziz Sheikh
© 2014 John Wiley & Sons, Ltd. Published 2014 by John Wiley & Sons, Ltd.

Introduction

Healthcare improvement aims to improve outcomes for patients by encouraging the adoption of improvement interventions that have solid evidence of effectiveness. However, in healthcare, in a review of 34 evidence-based interventions that had been replicated in other settings, 41% were found to have a smaller effect size or were not found to be effective. There is, therefore, some uncertainty around how best to adopt and implement new interventions.

Improvement initiatives when first established can be effective, but as they became more widespread, a diminishing effect on outcomes can be seen. One explanation (Figure 25.1) is that the effectiveness of an intervention is often based on studies in a small number of settings. The complexity of the intervention may not be fully understood before it is spread to another hospital or setting. For example, the 'Keystone ICU project' (described in Chapter 18) where intensive care units in Michigan, USA, reduced central venous catheter bloodstream infections by introducing technical interventions (changes in clinical practice) and non-technical interventions (linked to leadership, teamwork and culture change), has not always been successfully replicated elsewhere. Existing research suggests this is because the complexity of the intervention may not be fully understood. In this situation, a simple but intuitively appealing summary model of the changes needed to produce improvement becomes a fixed protocol rather than the basis of multiple plan–do–study–act (PDSA) cycles for teams to adapt the interventions locally. Local adaptation could permit understanding about the training needs of different staff groups and identify key clinical and managerial processes that would need to be in place for the intervention to be successful.

There is a risk of rushing to generate a summary of the changes needed to produce improvement outcomes too quickly, without truly understanding which change(s) led to improvement. In healthcare improvement, a promising new intervention (or change model) can be found to be effective in a small number of settings, but when replicated as a fixed protocol across a broad range of contexts, it is found to be ineffective. One way in which the improvement field aims to address such issues is by encouraging the small-scale testing of new changes, first in a small number of settings and then in an increasingly wide variety of settings.

Innovation phase

All new models of care have to originate from somewhere, and in improvement this can be referred to as the *innovation phase* (Figure 25.2). Typically, in this phase, a new model of care (or intervention) may have been developed in one or two settings. For example, a university teaching hospital may have developed and implemented a checklist aimed at ensuring that a number of evidence-based procedures are followed prior to a hip replacement. The innovation phase may aim to understand what impact the intervention has on patient outcomes and to describe the main changes that lead to improvement so that others can adapt it to their setting. There may be some evidence that the intervention is effective in this single setting, but it may not be clear whether it will be applicable or effective in many other settings.

Testing phase

The *testing phase* is used to help understand where an intervention can be adopted to work elsewhere. In this phase, improvement methods such as the Model for Improvement and PDSA cycles are used to undertake small tests of applying the new intervention in new settings. It is expected that improvement teams will undertake a number of PDSA cycles, adapting components of the intervention in order to learn whether or not it will work for them. The number of settings will increase and the types of settings will widen as evidence builds. For example, other university teaching hospitals may test the new model as well as non-academic, rural hospitals or hospitals with a different patient case mix from the original setting.

Problems can occur if the testing phase is not well conducted in a wide variety of settings, or is not undertaken at all. For example, if a hospital system decides to scale up a checklist based on evidence obtained from a single setting in the innovation phase, they may not have fully identified the key components of the intervention, and it may be that the checklist approach is only effective for certain patients in certain settings. Implementing the intervention across a wide variety of settings is likely to lead to poor overall effectiveness, resistant surgical staff and little if any sustained improvement in patient outcomes (see Figure 25.1).

Scale-up and spread phase

The *scale-up and spread phase* aims to broaden implementation. *Scale-up* occurs when there is a deliberate effort to push out or implement a new model on a long-term basis, across a particular system, in order to achieve sustained improvement in patient outcomes. For example, a large hospital system may aim to implement a surgical checklist across all component hospitals. To do so, hospital leaders may hope to bring about sustained improvement by introducing policy changes requiring action by surgical teams as well as midlevel and senior clinical managers. *Spread* may occur when other settings wish to replicate the new model. For example, hospitals may have heard or read about a new surgical checklist associated with improved patient outcomes, and they may decide to try to introduce the checklist in their setting.

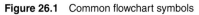

26 Quality improvement tools: visualisation

Figure 26.1 Common flowchart symbols

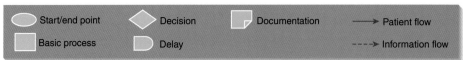

Figure 26.2 Example of a swim lane process map

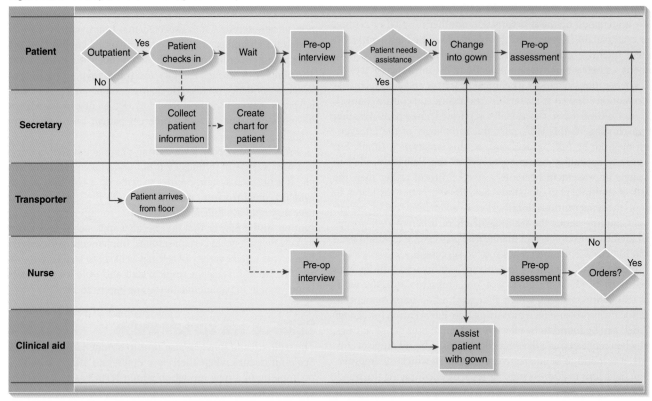

Figure 26.3 Example of a detailed swim lane process map for the day of surgery

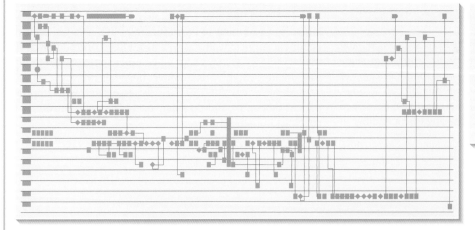

When blown up to be something you could actually read, this swim lane process map is 12 feet long and 3 feet high! It details how each stakeholder contributes to a surgical procedure, including how the patient and information move throughout the day. All process maps certainly do not require this level of detail (see Chapter 36 for a worked example in surgery)

Table 26.1 A suppliers, inputs, processes, outputs and customers (SIPOC) diagram template

Suppliers	Inputs	Process	Outputs	Customers
List suppliers here	List inputs here	Include process map or list the processes here	List outputs here	List customers here

Patient Safety and Healthcare Improvement at a Glance, First Edition. Edited by Sukhmeet S. Panesar, Andrew Carson-Stevens, Sarah A. Salvilla and Aziz Sheikh
© 2014 John Wiley & Sons, Ltd. Published 2014 by John Wiley & Sons, Ltd.

Introduction

Developing a better understanding of a process – rather than just your own tasks – is critical to improving quality and patient safety. This type of systems thinking is applicable beyond formal improvement work and can help clinicians to focus on healthcare quality continuously. A process map is a quality improvement tool to graphically represent steps in a process, and it helps everyone on the team to be sure that they understand the flow, delays, tasks and responsibilities associated with that process. An incomplete picture of a process is like looking at a portion of a painting with a magnifying glass without seeing what the whole painting actually depicts.

Creating a process map of the current system can help you to understand the process you are seeking to improve: how it works, who is involved and how it flows. It is also a useful visual aid for communicating the process to others who do not understand your process. Flowchart symbols (see Figure 26.1) are used to represent the sequence and flow of events throughout a process.

There are multiple approaches for building process maps – the actual state, the intended state or the ideal state – and it is sometimes helpful to consider more than one of these. If you want to map what is actually occurring (the actual state), you need to directly observe the process as the map is being created. What you observe can often be different from what people think is (or should be) happening, and therefore the intended and actual process maps may differ from one another.

Creating a process map

1. Determine the scope of the process to be mapped

Choose a specific starting point (a process trigger) and a specific ending point. The starting and ending points are critical to avoid 'scope creep', where the process map slowly grows to become unmanageable. It may not be effective to develop a process map of a patient's entire length of stay using a trigger of admission and an endpoint of discharge – that would be a very large process map! However, it could be helpful to map the patient experience during preoperative activities on the day of surgery to examine how the surgeon, anaesthesiologist, nurses and nurse anaesthetist interact with the patient. Additionally, the level of specificity is an important component of 'scope creep' as the map can get very large if the process to be mapped is complex. For example, entering patient data into the patient's notes may be considered a single process block (e.g. 'enter patient data'), or each data element could be considered a separate task (e.g. 'enter allergies' and 'enter medications').

2. Identify all of the stakeholders who have an effect on the process

Choose representatives from the stakeholder groups – those directly or indirectly involved in the process flow or outcomes – to help you develop the process map. It may not be feasible to have everyone involved in the process work together on the map, but observations and interviews can help fill in process activities. This activity can help to resolve misunderstandings about what is actually occurring in a process.

3. Have everyone on the team list the individual steps in the process

It is helpful to have stakeholders brainstorm and list all of the steps first, without focusing on the actual sequence of events. If each member of the team writes each individual step on a sticky note or index card, then the entire group can sort through and sequence the steps on a wall or table.

4. Work as a team to agree on the actual sequence of events and the appropriate flowchart symbols

While you are working together, it is almost certain that you will generate possible solutions that could better the process that you are trying to understand. Your focus now is on creating the map, but be sure to document these ideas. In addition, you should document any assumptions you use.

5. Share your map with all stakeholders and make edits or additions as necessary

Allow stakeholders to comment on your drafts, especially if they were not involved in its creation. Their insights can help clarify and refine the process map. Healthcare processes are complex, and everyone might not agree on the current state process map. This is an opportunity to identify areas for improvement or clarity.

Additional details

A swim lane process map has an additional level of detail: 'lanes' guide the alignment of the steps in the map to visually represent who is responsible for certain aspects of the process (Figures 26.2 and 26.3). This type of process map may be particularly useful to illustrate patient or information handoffs.

A suppliers, inputs, processes, outputs and customers (SIPOC) diagram (Table 26.1) can help you frame a process map by first listing these additional elements. For example, consider the process depicted in Figure 26.2. To determine what to map, it may be helpful to consider the different providers (e.g. surgeon, anaesthesia provider and circulating nurse) who supply inputs to the preoperative process (interviews, orders for additional tests etc.). Lab results, completed forms and other outputs are necessary before the patient and surgical team (the 'customers') can proceed to surgery. Once you've considered the suppliers, inputs, outputs, and customers, it may be much easier to create the actual process map of more complex systems.

27 Quality improvement: assessing the system

Table 27.1 Failure modes and effects analysis (FMEA) template

Potential failure modes	Possible causes	Probability of occurrence	Failure effect	Severity of effect	Detection method	Ease of detection	Risk priority number
List the ways your system can potentially fail here	List potential causes for each of the failure modes here	Assign a score (1–10) for each of the failure modes	List what happens when each of the failures occur	Assign a score (1–10) for each of the failure effects	How do you currently know when the failure has occurred?	Assign a score (1–10) for how easily failures are detected	Multiply the probability of occurrence, severity of effect, and ease of detection scores

Figure 27.1 Sample failure modes and effects analysis (FMEA) for potential failures to the magnetic resonance imaging (MRI) schedule from a patient arriving late to their appointment

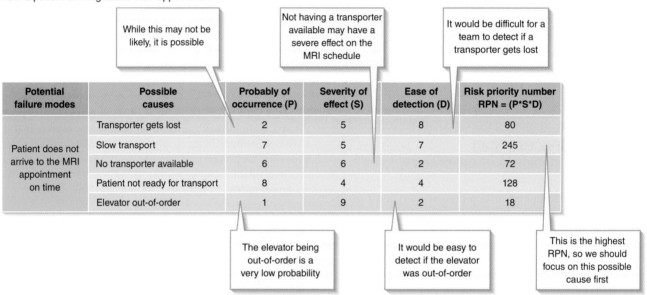

Figure 27.2 Sample fishbone diagram for late surgical procedures at the start of each day

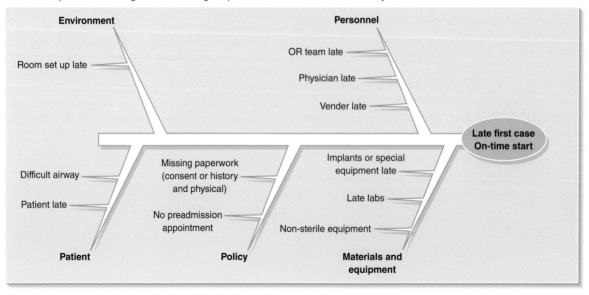

Patient Safety and Healthcare Improvement at a Glance, First Edition. Edited by Sukhmeet S. Panesar, Andrew Carson-Stevens, Sarah A. Salvilla and Aziz Sheikh
© 2014 John Wiley & Sons, Ltd. Published 2014 by John Wiley & Sons, Ltd.

Evaluating your process

Once a process map has been created, it can facilitate multiple strategies to evaluate potential failures, errors and breakdowns in the process. Two of these approaches are the failure modes and effects analysis (FMEA) and the why-why approach. Generally these brainstorming techniques do not generate solutions to issues, but rather serve as a means to identify and preliminarily prioritise potential quality improvement (QI) areas.

Processes are designed to work a certain way. When processes do not function optimally, they may contain potential opportunities for system failures. Even if a patient is not harmed, a process breakdown could still be a considered a system failure. The two tools described below can be used to identify potential causes of a process breakdown.

Failure Modes and Effects Analysis

The purpose of FMEA is to *preemptively* examine potential opportunities for your system or process to fail, generate errors or break down, and, through a structured approach, prioritise improvement projects to address these potential failures. FMEA is not generally used as a reactive tool as its purpose is to help identify potential failures before they occur.

Once you identify an opportunity to use FMEA, choose a team that represents your stakeholders. There are several variations on the FMEA method. We recommend the FMEA template shown in Table 27.1 to organise your brainstorming and guide the assignment of priorities for improvement opportunities using the following steps:

1 **With the team, brainstorm all of the ways your process could fail.** Each process in the process map (see Chapter 26) can fail if it does not do what it is intended to do.

2 **For each of the process breakdowns you identify in step 1, list all of the potential causes that could contribute to that failure.** This is where you consider how a failure could happen. Consider all of the potential causes for each of the potential failures, but note that there could be overlap.

3 **Estimate the probability of occurrence for each of the potential causes you identify in step 2.** Assign a score of 1–10, where 1 represents something that is not very likely to occur and 10 represents something that will almost certainly occur.

4 **For each of the causes you identify in step 2, consider the effect of the failure as well as the severity of that effect.** List what happens when failures occur, and assign a score of 1–10 to represent the severity of the occurrence. Lower scores represent an outcome that presents very little risk, where a score of 10 represents the most severe outcome.

5 **Consider the current methods to detect when a failure has occurred.** What methods, controls or warnings are in place that would help you and your teams identify when a failure has occurred? Assign a score of 1–10, where 1 represents something that you would almost certainly detect and a score of 10 indicates a failure that is surely unlikely to be noticed.

6 *Calculate a risk priority number (RPN) by multiplying the probability of occurrence, severity of effect and ease of detection scores.*

For several of the tasks above, the user assigns a score from 1 to 10 ranking the probability of occurrence, severity of the failure and ease of detection. There is diversity in the QI literature about how each score should be selected and operationalised, and often in the healthcare setting, a 1–5 scale is used. The most important thing is that you and your team are consistent in how you select these scores. Very simply, lower scores indicate lower probabilities of occurrence, lower probabilities of severity and greater ease of detection. For example, Figure 27.1 is a basic example of an FMEA but demonstrates how scores can be selected for specific causes.

Potential causes with the RPNs should become high-priority improvement initiatives for you and your team. However, certain potential causes should be given highest priority. You should think carefully about the limits of severity scores and occurrence rates; generally, experts recommend prioritising failure modes with severity scores of 7–10 and events that can occur very frequently.

Why-why approach

A why-why analysis is used to identify root causes that may lead to potential failures, errors and breakdowns in processes. Ask each QI team member to reflect on why a potential problem could occur. This will likely lead to multiple ideas, and for each of these continue to ask, 'Why?' until a potential root cause has been identified. Typically, asking 'Why?' five times will elucidate a potential root cause (hence this is sometimes called the '5 Whys analysis'). The results can also be displayed in a fishbone diagram (named for its overall shape), shown in Figure 27.2, where the overall effect is listed at the 'head' of the fish. The large bones are used to classify possible cause categories, typically identified as personnel, environment, policies, patients and materials and equipment. Each large bone can be divided into smaller bones representing sub-classifications of potential causes.

Other tools

Understanding the processes and potential causes for problems is the first step in quality improvement. The next steps in quality improvement use statistical tools to quantify, evaluate and monitor improvement and are not discussed here.

28 Patient stories in improvement

Figure 28.1 Summary of the process for collecting patient stories

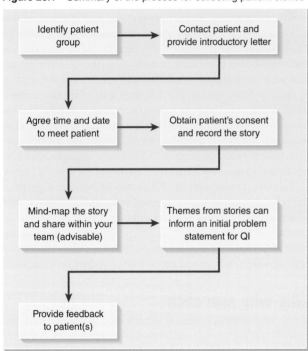

	Tips for mind-mapping
1.	Take a large, blank, landscape page of paper (i.e. turn the page so you can use the full width of the paper)
2.	In the centre of the page place the name, identifying code or alias of your patient, thus representing the subject of your mind map
3.	Use words and illustrations/drawings throughout your map. Wherever possible use single keywords in the early stages, circling them to ensure they are clearly visible. Each keyword should be written along its own line (known as a branch)
4.	When a keyword is identified, make a note of the timing this occurred during the audio/video recording. This will assist you and your colleagues to re-listen to this section of the story again
5.	Once you have completed listening and mind-mapping the story, listen to the whole story again, adding more details to the key words that were initially plotted
6.	See if there are connections between words. If so, draw a line between them to make the association between emerging ideas as clear as possible
7.	Experiment with different ways of linking and elaborating aspects of the patient's story – use highlighters, codes and arrows
8.	This process should be repeated until the map represents the totality of the story

Figure 28.2 An example of a patient story mind map

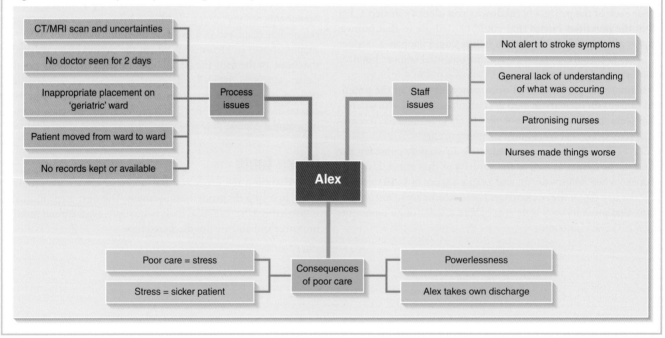

Introduction

For centuries, stories have been told through the media of talk, writing or graphics. Stories are a valuable means of communication between humans. However, with increasing value being attributed to objective scientific knowledge in recent decades, stories (which are by nature more subjective) have been somewhat overlooked as a resource for improving the quality of healthcare. Nevertheless, this situation is beginning to change. The UK NHS, for example, has recently taken steps to ensure the experiences of its patients, as well as those close to them such as family members, are listened to.

When patient stories are skillfully collected and utilised, they enable the health service to better understand what is working well and areas where patient and carer experience can be improved. As such, patient stories may become 'mobilising narratives' that help inspire healthcare teams to improve their service.

The process of collecting patient stories

The process of collecting patient stories follows a series of steps (see Figure 28.1). Key steps are considered in this process:
- Recruiting patients and obtaining consent
- Ethically conducting and recording the story
- Making sense of the story – mind mapping

Recruit patients and obtain consent

It is important to contact potential storytellers who have recently experienced the service or patient journey you are aiming to improve. It may be tempting to only collect stories from patients who are easy to access and communicate with, while excluding patients with whom communication or access is more difficult. However, collecting stories from only one group of patients will not provide a fair picture of patient experience, and bias may be introduced into the project.

Stories should not be recorded unless storytellers are informed and provide valid written consent beforehand. All information that is necessary to storytellers to enable truly informed consent must be given in advance. Storytellers should be asked to sign a *consent form*, which will allow the use of the final version of the story as a publicly available learning resource that aims to improve the quality of healthcare.

Ethically conduct and record the story

There are three practical ethical behaviours that should be displayed at all times when working with a patient story:
- **Respect:** Storytellers and their stories should be treated with respect at all times. The intentions of the storyteller will be interpreted accurately, thus preserving the integrity of the story
- **Support:** Storytellers will be offered emotional support during and after telling their stories
- **Confidentiality and anonymity:** Remind storytellers not to name other patients or staff members during the story. All

information collected from patients is to be kept in such a way that protects their identity unless they wish to be identified, as many do.

The process of collecting the story involves good communication skills that help the patient to feel at ease when recounting experiences. Establishing trust and rapport with the patient is important. For example, practising the opening introduction of the interview will help you confidently explain to the patient why you are undertaking the project, in a manner that will reassure the patient but also establish trust and rapport. Now is also a good time to explain to the storyteller that stories are audio-recorded or (sometimes) video-recorded, thus ensuring that attention can be paid to listening rather than making notes. Recording also ensures accurate recall and allows the story to be listened to repeatedly with others in the team and beyond (N.B. ensure that patients consent to their stories being shared with others).

Following the introduction, the interaction moves to a series of questions about the patient's experiences. The aim here is to allow the patient to speak as freely as possible within the time allocated. Therefore, open questions should largely be used that will encourage patients to recollect and expand on their experiences. Closed or probing questions are justified when specific information or clarification is required. However, closed-type questions require caution and skill if the patient is not to feel rushed, or the conversation seems perfunctory rather than genuinely participative.

It is generally unavoidable that, at certain times, you will need to add structure or direction to the interaction. However, in between these times, the patient will greatly value the experience of being listened to. Active listening is one of the most important ingredients for successfully collecting stories. During active listening, attentiveness is demonstrated to the speaker through a variety of actions, for example maintaining eye contact with the speaker or nodding at certain times to demonstrate understanding or that a certain point has been noted.

Making sense of the story – mind mapping

To ensure that patient stories lead to improvements in healthcare, it is imperative that the key components of the story are disseminated to colleagues. It is impractical to expect staff to read a whole patient story or even a lengthy précis of the story. Instead, the story should be summarised into the main learning or analytical themes, which are then used as themes and triggers for future service improvements.

A mind-mapping approach is often used as a means of transforming the totality of the story into a condensed graphical representation (see Figure 28.2 for a worked example). To make sense of the story, you should play back the recording of each story and 'mind map' the contents. The mind map should offer a means of reducing the totality of a story into main themes that can then be compared with the stories of other patients (see the 'Tips for mind mapping' box for more details).

29 Leading change in healthcare

Figure 29.1 25 reasons to change

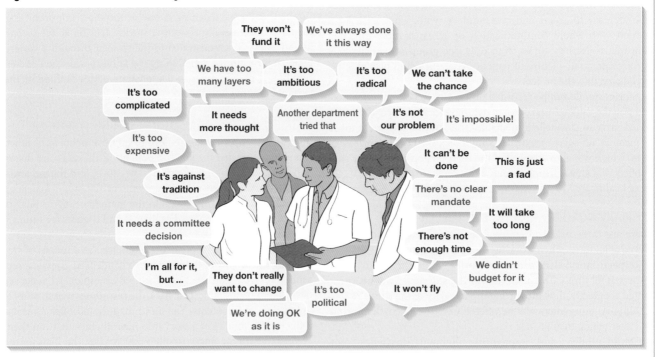

Source: Adapted from a presentation slide given by patient safety leaders at WellStar Health System, USA

Figure 29.2 25 reasons not to change

Source: Adapted from Bumsted P. Biocultural Science and Management; http://13c4.wordpress.com/2007/02/24/50-reasons-not-to-change/

Patient Safety and Healthcare Improvement at a Glance, First Edition. Edited by Sukhmeet S. Panesar, Andrew Carson-Stevens, Sarah A. Salvilla and Aziz Sheikh.
© 2014 John Wiley & Sons, Ltd. Published 2014 by John Wiley & Sons, Ltd.

Opposing the status quo

Leading improvements in healthcare can be challenging. However, once you start, you are likely to spend the rest of your career seeking to improve the systems that lead to poor patient experience and harm. Becoming a 'radical' against existing systems is not just about speaking up when bad things happen (which is very important), but also about taking action in your own area of influence to make high-quality care the norm. A radical is a courageous, passionate person who is willing to challenge the status quo and take responsibility for change.

Figure 29.1 provides a powerful visual of the consequences of poor-quality healthcare and can be the catalyst for involving others in your ideas for change. Looking at the history of change and improvement, big change only happens in organisations because of radicals. However, there are many forces opposing the changes you will want to see. For example: systems that reward their workers for 'keeping the trains running' rather than seeking ways to improve care; people in powerful positions who have a vested interest in keeping the status quo; and colleagues and leaders who are sceptical, apathetic or scared of change (Figure 29.2).

So who are the most effective radicals in healthcare organisations? Research by organisational behaviour expert Debra Meyerson suggests that the people who get the best outcomes from change are those who have learnt to oppose and conform at the same time. Or, as she puts it, 'They are able to rock the boat and yet stay in it'. These are the champions for change who stand up to challenge the existing order of things when they see there could be a better way. They develop the ability to walk the fine line between difference and fit, inside and outside. These leaders are driven by their own convictions and values, which makes them credible and authentic to others in their organisations. Most importantly of all, they take action as individuals who, by involving others, ignite the kind of broader collective action that leads to big change.

Characteristics of radicals

Radicals already exist in every healthcare organisation, in many different roles and at many different levels. They are not typically the chief executives or senior clinical leaders, yet the impact of their change activities is often just as significant.

Successful leaders often invest time and effort building effective networks and relationships with others; continuously seek innovative new ways of delivering care and reducing harm; and commit to the patient-centred mission and values of the healthcare organisation they work for. They are driven by a passion for better, safer care for patients; are optimistic about the future and the potential for change; see many possibilities for doing things in different ways; and generate energy for change which attracts others to collaborate with them for the shared common cause of better quality healthcare.

'Troublemakers' also challenge the way things stand but in a different manner to that of radicals. Troublemakers complain about the current state of affairs, but their focus tends to be around their own personal position rather than achieving the goals of the organisation. Troublemakers are angry about how things are and do not have much confidence that things will get better in the future. They alienate other people because if others link with them, troublemakers will sap their energy.

Figure 29.3 contrasts the characteristics of radicals and troublemakers.

Surviving as a radical

There are a few challenges for improvement leaders in this radical–troublemaker distinction. Firstly, many organisational leaders view anyone who challenges the status quo as a troublemaker. Therefore, radicals can get unfairly labelled as troublemakers when they challenge existing systems and processes that create the potential for poor-quality care. Sometimes, this has the impact of making potential radicals keep quiet or conform when the most appropriate action would be to take action or speak up. Secondly, lots of people who care deeply about high-quality healthcare start out as radicals, but their voice does not get heard or they are ignored or ridiculed. As a result, they can begin to noisily question the status quo in an antagonistic and self-defeating manner, and eventually cross the line from radical to troublemaker.

History shows us that troublemaker tactics are hardly ever likely to get the results sought. As an improvement leader, you have a responsibility to watch out for this in your own behaviours and try to prevent it from happening by building relationships and forming alliances with others who are also willing to stand up and be counted for better patient care.

Figure 29.3 Comparing the characteristics of radicals and troublemakers

Troublemaker	Radical
Complain	Create
Me focused	Mission focused
Anger	Passion
Pessimist	Optimist
Energy sapping	Energy generating
Alienate	Attract
Problems	Possibilities
Alone	Together

Figure 29.4 Being a great change agent is about knowing, doing, living and being improvement

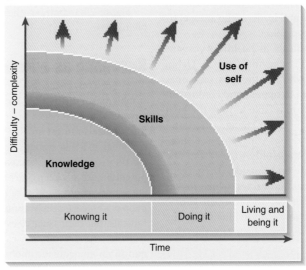

Box 29.1 Some calls to action for improvement leaders leaders as healthcare radicals

1.	Make time to reflect on your own role as a healthcare improvement leader; what are the implications for acting as an agent or leader of change?
2.	Seek out other radicals who share your mission and discuss tactics for rocking the boat and staying in it
3.	Identify and support others who are at risk of crossing the line from 'rebel' to 'troublemaker'
4.	Think about how you adopt or build the 'spirit of the student' and how your role as an active learner can be a catalyst for others
5.	Reflect on the extent to which you are knowing, doing, living and being healthcare improvement and patient safety; to what extent are you operating from your true self? How can you make your impact as a healthcare radical even more effective?

Box 29.2 Key messages for leading change

1.	Big change only happens in healthcare organisations because of the courageous people ('radicals, rebels, dissenters and heretics') who **show there can be a different and better future**
2.	Being a healthcare improvement leader inevitably means **challenging the status quo of how systems and processes of patient care are organised**
3.	Walk the fine line between difference and fit, inside and outside, conformity and rebellion; those who can **rock the boat and stay in it are most successful**
4.	**Change yourself first**, rather than just expecting other people to change
5.	Adopt 'the spirit of the student' – be open to **continuous learning, embrace new ideas and approaches and be willing to challenge and change your own beliefs**
6.	It is important (but insufficient) to build knowledge and skills in improvement; to be truly effective as a leader, you have to **be a role model for everyone else**

How to be a radical: start close to home first

Learning the methods and tools for delivering high-quality patient care will give you a new set of eyes for looking at the healthcare system. Whatever clinical setting you work in, you will be able to look at the world around you and see things that need improving; the medication process that should be reconciled, the preoperative system that creates the risk of infection or the labelling system which might lead to a drug error. However, if you are going to be a truly effective improvement leader, starting your own self-improvement work at an even earlier point is essential. Do not be tempted to launch into big efforts to influence other people to change the way they currently think and work, before reflecting on and changing your own practices first. This is well understood by David Whyte when he says, 'I do not think you can really deal with change without a person asking real questions about who they are and how they belong in the world'.

Improvement leaders are signal generators, and their words and deeds are constantly scrutinised and interpreted by the people around them in different teams and departments. The amplification effect of what was done and said is far greater than we can imagine. Thus, perhaps the most powerful way to inspire others to change is to be the role model for that change. If you want other people to take a risk and change the way they think or carry out their roles for healthcare improvement, you have to take the lead. As Tanveer Naseer describes it:

> *You have to be the first one up and off the high dive you're asking others to leap from. Ask yourself: where am I playing it too safe and what is that safety costing me? Then leap from your platform of safety into the cold water of change.*

By taking action, the most effective radicals are able to achieve small wins that create bigger ripples in the organisation, building a sense of hope and confidence that it is possible to make a difference. They can then join forces with others who are also committed to the cause, working as a collective force for changes that are commonly valued.

So, as an improvement leader, you should create your own goals for change, work out how and where to make a contribution to the bigger cause, seek and reach out to build alliances with others and demonstrate the will to move the change agenda forward. When you have the courage to act proactively like this, most line managers and leaders will value these behaviours, even where the organisation does not currently have a strong quality improvement culture.

Generating signals for success

Fear is a major inhibitor of improvement leadership. People can be afraid to challenge or report poor-quality care because of fear of repercussion or reprisal. Fear is also a significant barrier to learning – it is hard to learn when you feel fear. An improvement culture requires people to move away from a status quo that they feel comfortable with and into a brave new world of quality control (standardisation of procedures based on evidence-based practice), quality improvement (thinking about healthcare in terms of the six aims of quality and more) and quality planning (realising the steps needed to translate the quality improvement policy agenda into workable actions in the workplace), and that can be scary. As Peter Senge wrote in *The Fifth Discipline*:

> *When we see that to learn we must be willing to look foolish, to let another teach us, learning doesn't always look so good anymore.... Only with the support and fellowship of another can we face the dangers of learning meaningful things.*

This situation creates a specific call to action for healthcare radicals. As a signal generator at the leading edge of change, you must embrace the spirit of the student. This means taking responsibility for your own learning and being open to continuous learning, embracing new ideas and approaches and being willing to challenge and change your existing belief systems. Your learning must move beyond knowledge and skills. For radicals, it is important, but not enough, to continuously build your knowledge of improvement methods and approaches. It is also important, but not enough, to take responsibility for your own development as a skilled leader or a facilitator of change. What sets healthcare radicals apart is the extent to which they purposefully seek to 'live' and 'be' improvement in the way they operate in the world and in their interactions and relationships with others. Figure 29.4 captures the relationship of those competencies.

History also teaches that organisational or system transformation is always preceded by personal transformation. So if, as a healthcare radical, you want to play your role in radical changes for patient safety, you should focus deeply on your own perspective and the ways you interact with and influence others. Chapter 30 explores the role of narrative in public leadership; consider how you can use storytelling to radically involve others in your vision for change.

The more people you can influence in a positive way, the more that you and your followers (as organisational radicals) can unleash a powerful reservoir of energy for change, and the more difference you can collectively make for your patients.

30 Public narrative: story of self, us and now

Figure 30.1 Story of self, story of now and story of us

Story of self
Call to leadership

Purpose

Story of now
Strategy and action

Community

Story of us
Shared values and
shared experience

Urgency

Source: Adapted with permission from Professor Marshall Ganz, Harvard University, Boston, MA, USA

Challenge

- What was the specific challenge you faced?

Choice

- What was the specific choice you made?
- Why?
- How did it make you feel?

Outcome

- What happened?
- What hope does it give us?
- Whay do you want to teach us?
- How do you want us to feel?

Introduction

Stories can be powerful tools to inspire others to work with you to change existing practices. Social organisers – those who rally people towards shared common goals – use 'public narrative' as a method for cultivating the hearts and minds of those who can help to bring about change. Having a 'public narrative' to encourage others to work with you can be useful for building a team and gaining momentum to achieve your vision for change.

Public narrative has three elements: a story of why you personally believe a change is needed now – *a story of self*; a story of why you think those listening might believe a change is needed too – *a story of us*; and a story of what makes the challenge ahead so urgent to act upon – *a story of now* (see how the three elements connect in Figure 30.1).

Story of self

Telling a 'story of self' is a way to share the values that define who you are based on your lived experiences. This can be made up of choice points, which are moments when you have faced a challenge (e.g. the decision to speak out when you've seen a problem in care), made a choice (e.g. the act of speaking up), experienced a positive or negative outcome (e.g. how those around you reacted and what they said) or learned a moral (e.g. speaking up for a patient when everyone else was ignoring her). Think about challenge, choice and outcome in your own story. The outcome might be what you learned in addition to what happened. Powerful stories leave your listeners with images in their minds that

shape their understanding of you and your calling. Articulating the decisions you make in the face of challenges ultimately communicates your values.

> *Elizabeth is a 79-year-old woman who was admitted for investigations to try to explain her chest pain. Before the weekend, she was full of life and had a smile from ear to ear on the ward round. Today, she wasn't smiling. She was wincing in pain and appeared confused. She had fallen on Saturday night by tripping over her telemetry leads. I was distraught by the fact we couldn't ensure the safety of a patient who was in good health before her admission and now has a broken hip and is at a higher risk of mortality. Our team missed the opportunity to discontinue her telemetry before the weekend.*

Story of Us

The purpose of the 'story of us' is to bring alive the values your audience shares with each other that can inspire collective action. Your goal is to tell a story that (1) evokes shared values that can unite the group, (2) highlight the challenge(s) faced that makes action urgent, and (3) give hope that, if you work together a specific change is possible. If your team is developing a quality improvement intervention, then you must think of it in that context. What are the shared values of your team and those you are trying to engage?

The 'story of us' draws upon the values and shared experiences of the group. It becomes a moral resource (or a reminder of why change was needed) and can be called upon as the group moves

Patient Safety and Healthcare Improvement at a Glance, First Edition. Edited by Sukhmeet S. Panesar, Andrew Carson-Stevens, Sarah A. Salvilla and Aziz Sheikh
© 2014 John Wiley & Sons, Ltd. Published 2014 by John Wiley & Sons, Ltd.

forwards to face uncertainty. Stories of us can inspire, teach, offer hope and advise caution. They can shift power relationships ('We're all in this together') to build new communities of passionate people committed to making change happen.

Our team had a meeting about how this could be avoided. I remember for the last 6 months, nurses have been asking us during the middle of the day, 'Can we remove the urinary catheter?' and 'Can we remove the telemetry?' As a junior doctor, we addressed the issue at that time or deferred it for a later time. In the meantime, we increase the risk of adverse events if the patient doesn't need either. We had weekly conversations as a result that asked questions of how we could minimise errors, avoid interruptions, improve quality and decrease costs as they relate to telemetry and urinary catheters. Together, we created a review system that we would run with each patient at the conclusion of each encounter; we would ask about the need for telemetry, catheters, in fact any unnecessary attachment or intrusion on the patient. If they didn't need them, we would discontinue them and the nurses would remove them. Using the Model for Improvement, we learned how to adapt the concept with other medical teams and eventually spread this across all the medical teams in the hospital.

Story of Now

The story of now must articulate an urgent challenge that the community (now known as the 'us') shares. Here, story and strategy overlap because a key element in hope is a theory of change – a credible vision of how to get from A to Z. A meaningful choice is more like 'We all must choose – do we commit to improving care until catheter-related infections are zero or not?' A vision can begin by getting a number of people to show up at a meeting that you committed to run. You can achieve a 'small' victory that shows change is possible. A small victory can become a source of hope if it is interpreted as part of a greater vision.

In a public hospital where we are strapped for resources and inspired to provide the best care possible for our patients, simple interventions make a difference. Six months later, the rate of inpatient falls is down by 20%, the infection rate is down 5% and we have saved the healthcare system thousands of pounds. These results got the attention of other junior doctors on the sidelines. As we continued to tell our story, others joined. Our efforts moved from telemetry and catheters to cancelled blood results, health education, improved medicines reconciliation and redesigning surgical pre-assessment clinics. We were becoming a beacon of hope for high-quality patient-centred care.

Conclusion

The narratives are linked. The *now* is linked to *self* through the purpose for which the authority will call upon others to join in action. The story of *now* creates urgency rooted in the values shared by the *us* who one hopes to move. The goal is not to have a final 'script'. The goal is to learn a process by which you can generate your narrative, and call upon it, when, where and how you need to in order to motivate yourself and others to purposeful action.

31 Planning an improvement project

Figure 31.1 An overview of planning an improvement project

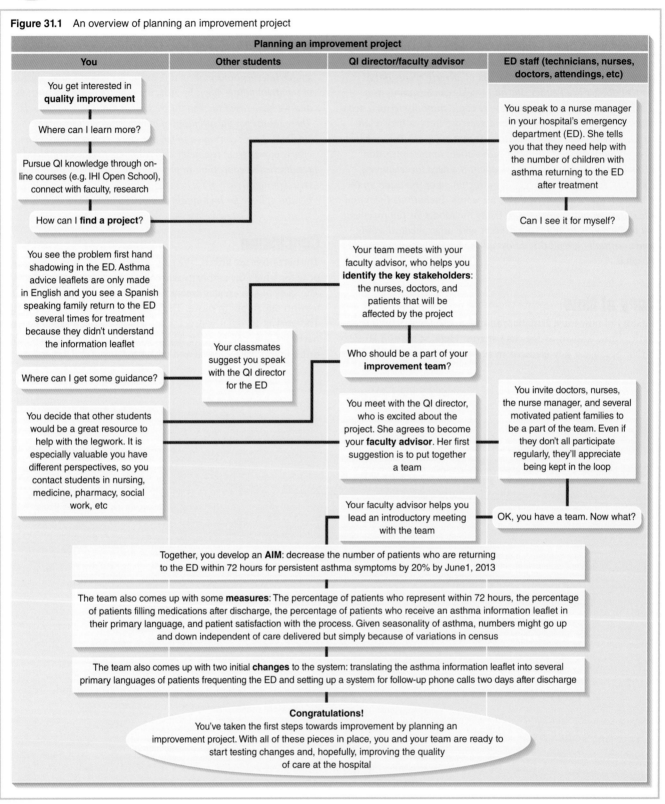

Patient Safety and Healthcare Improvement at a Glance, First Edition. Edited by Sukhmeet S. Panesar, Andrew Carson-Stevens, Sarah A. Salvilla and Aziz Sheikh
© 2014 John Wiley & Sons, Ltd. Published 2014 by John Wiley & Sons, Ltd.

Introduction

There are seven important steps to getting started on a successful quality improvement project (see Figure 31.1):

1 Learn about quality improvement.
2 Find a project.
3 Form a team.
4 Find a faculty advisor.
5 Identify the key stakeholders.
6 Develop an aim and measures.
7 Identify changes.

Learn about quality improvement

See Chapters 21–27.

Find a project

There are several ways you could identify a quality improvement project, including:

1 Drawing on experiences as a student (or even if you've spent time as a patient); you might have observed things that did not work as well as they should have. Did patients have to wait for a long time before they are seen in a clinic? Was there a lack of communication between physicians and nurses at the bedside?
2 Talk to people who work in healthcare organisations. Frontline staff who take care of patients every day know which systems work well and which need improving. Ask them what they think is wrong. Or ask them what one thing they would improve if they could.
3 Routinely ask patients during your interaction, "What can I do to improve your stay?" Ask enough patients and it is likely that potential themes for improvement will emerge.
4 Identify and talk with those in charge of care quality in specific clinical areas – directors of quality, nurse managers or clinical directors. Staff members in these leadership positions often manage a number of ongoing projects that strive to improve care for patients. You could join one of these projects and learn from experienced professionals about how to conduct quality improvement projects.

It is important to start small when beginning a quality improvement project. Do not try to improve the infection rates in the entire healthcare organisation. Start in one hospital, on one ward, at one bedside, with one patient. Use the Model for Improvement to determine what works, and then scale up.

Form a team

Collaboration is essential. Building a diverse group of team members working towards a shared common goal is integral to success. In quality improvement, teams do not comprise just one type of professional – reach out to other disciplines, including medicine, nursing, pharmacy, public health and even engineering. By having multiple disciplines, you can get a sense of how others view the healthcare system. And, through this broader perspective, you will be able to find bigger problems and better solutions.

Find a faculty advisor

It is critical to have someone who can advocate for you and your improvement team. This person may be the leader of a specific clinical team or a member of faculty at your university. He or she will provide active coaching throughout the process and facilitate connections with your local healthcare setting.

Identify the key stakeholders

Who is going to affect your project? And who is going to be affected by your project? Will you need to work with a certain physician? All the nurse educators? A few members of the pharmacy department? It is important to figure out this information as soon as possible and then contact the appropriate stakeholders early and often as you begin a project.

It might help to outline the stakeholders in your project using a simple 2×2 matrix (see Table 31.1).

Table 31.1 2×2 matrix for stakeholder analysis

	Low interest and involvement in process	High interest and involvement in process
High power and influence	*Satisfy*: Keep this group posted on important developments, and make sure they are satisfied at the end of the project.	*Engage*: Keep this group fully engaged from the start. They will be instrumental in making your project a success.
Low power and influence	*Monitor*: Keep an eye on this group, but realise that your time and resources might limit your interactions with it.	*Inform*: Keep this group well informed throughout the process, as they will be affected just as much as the group above.

Develop an aim and measures

Two mistakes that are often made when trying to improve a care process are starting a project without a goal and/or a measurement plan. A goal (or, in quality improvement terminology, an aim) tells you where you are going. It answers the first question in the Model for Improvement: 'What are we trying to accomplish?' An aim statement needs to be specific, measureable and actionable. Here is a bad aim statement: 'Our team wants to reduce medication errors'. Why is it bad? It is not specific and does not say how much, by when or for whom. Instead, say: 'Our team aims to decrease the number of medication errors by 20% for patients in the intensive care unit by 5 December 2015'.

Similarly, without an effective measurement plan (refer back to Chapter 24 for more detail), you will not know if your interventions are leading to improvement. This answers the second question in the Model for Improvement: 'How will we know that a change is an improvement?' Typically, improvement projects include outcome measures, process measures and balancing measures.

Identify changes

The last step before you start improving is coming up with some changes to test. In this stage, you will answer the question 'What changes can we make that will result in improvement?' For example, let us say you want to improve the percentage of patients who take their medications after a consultation. One change you might try is setting up a system to call them 2 days after they receive the prescription and remind them to take their medication.

32 Managing an improvement project

Figure 32.1 Initiating and executing a project plan

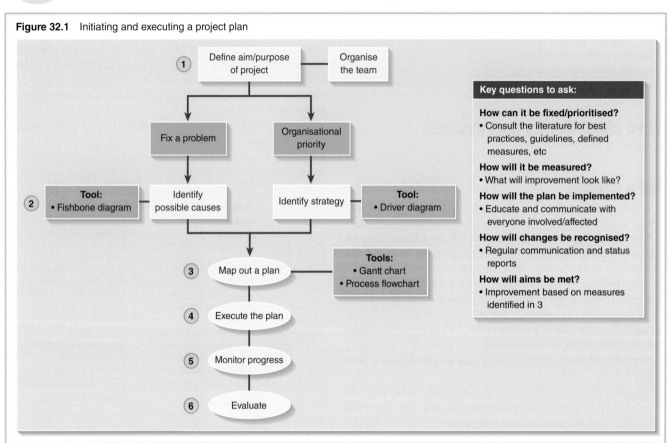

Introduction – developing strategies

In an industry where costs are growing and resources are constrained, good stewardship of healthcare is imperative. At the centre of activities to achieve better value for money are well-thought-out improvement projects that are successfully managed. Project management is the 'application of knowledge, skills, tools and techniques to project activities to meet the project requirements', often when the solutions to a problem are known. It is a strategy used in most industries. Managing healthcare improvement projects does not necessarily require knowledge and skills unique to healthcare, but the tools and techniques may differ from those used for project management in other fields. Improvement tools can be used when solutions are unknown and need to be developed or tested, for developing strategy and for monitoring progress towards the aim(s) of your project. Here, we consider how to merge best practices from project management (i.e. the role of the project manager) with the benefits of using improvement methods, to keep your improvement project on track.

Characteristics of a project

In healthcare, improvement projects are planned and evaluated using short cycles. Each cycle has a beginning and an end, it is based on a defined time period of learning, and the end point is determined by specific criteria related to an anticipated result. Projects develop as a result of a need to fix a problem or an organisational priority (Figure 32.1). Planning the amount of resources that will be required to complete a project is essential, and a comparison of costs and benefits helps project managers evaluate the feasibility of seeing the project through to completion.

A project typically develops out of a recognised need, whether it is to fix or to improve, although the approach is essentially the same (Figure 32.1, Steps 1 and 2). The key difference is that projects related to a problem must first investigate potential causes of the problem. A number of tools have been developed to work through this process (e.g. a fishbone diagram, as discussed in Chapter 27) and are described in the context of project planning. When a project develops out of an organisational priority, on the other hand, the focus turns towards information gathering – what have others done, what does the literature indicate as best practices and how do guidelines and performance measures help guide organisations focused on the same priority?

Once the project strategy is decided, a plan can be mapped out to clarify who will be responsible for each aspect of the project. Important considerations include what will be done, by whom, by when and how it will be measured to evaluate progress towards the aim (Figure 32.1, Step 3; the plan–do–study–act (PDSA) form in Chapter 23 and the 'Seven steps to measurement' in Chapter 24 are used here). Next, the project team implements the plan, giving consideration to how the people involved will be impacted (Step 4). For example, if the aim was to reduce readmissions and the team is implementing a strategy to follow up with patients within 24 hours of discharge, the hospital providers, discharge planners, cardiologists, general practitioners and patient, and any providers involved in the transition of that patient, would need to be aware of the new process and their role. Once the strategy is underway, it is critical to monitor it regularly (Step 5); a run chart (or Shewhart chart), as described in Chapter 24, can serve as a visual display and update. A chart should exist for each project-related measure.

Finally, progress towards the aim(s) (Step 1 using the Model for Improvement) must be evaluated. Improvement is continuous.

Step 6 helps determine what is working and reflecting on the team's belief in the changes and resulting improvements could be useful. Modifications could be needed to the next PDSA cycles. Steps 4–6 are your regular opportunities to take a bird's-eye view of your project to take stock of what has been achieved and what remains based on the changes you have developed and tested via PDSA cycles to date.

The role of the project manager

The project manager is responsible for organising, managing and holding accountable the involved parties. Successful management of an improvement project is related to the participants having a sense of ownership of the process that is developed and tested, the outcomes that result, and how promising change models are eventually implemented in practice and sustained. Management is not, however, the same as leadership when it comes to working with a team towards a successful outcome. 'Leader managers' set themselves apart from other managers; whilst their projects could be based in short time periods, leader managers think over the long term and ask: 'How will this project impact the future of the organisation, and will this project be the stepping-stone for other initiatives that have the potential to impact the organisation in the long term?' Such projects are also planned and executed with the interests of the organisation in mind, not simply a single aspect of the organisation without consideration given to others. And when organisational politics begin to challenge the project's impact, leader managers are equipped to manage the interests of multiple constituents. To that end, there is an emphasis placed on the vision and values of the organisation on the part of leader managers, and they by no means accept the status quo. Leader managers are focused on the aims of the project and leading a team towards successful outcomes.

Tools

A number of tools developed for project management and others focused on healthcare quality improvement are outlined in Table 32.1. Each of these tools serves a different purpose and can be useful at specific points in the project, from working to identify the cause of a problem, outlining the key steps in your project or mapping a timeline to ensure your project is completed in a timely fashion. When working to fix a problem, tools such as the fishbone diagram could be helpful to determine potential causes. If you were trying to improve a complex process like diabetic management, a process flowchart could be useful. To progress the learning from ideas elicited by those tools, a change model like the Model for Improvement will next help to keep track and make sense of the impact that the ideas and concepts (which you have identified from searching the literature or borrowing from elsewhere, or are developing and testing de novo) are having on achieving your goals.

A driver diagram is most useful when you have a specific aim in mind; that is, you know what you want to achieve (Figure 32.2). Let us continue with the example of diabetic management with the aim of HbA1c test results being available at the time of a patient visit. We need to explore the factors that may influence completing the test before an appointment, such as the doctor or nurse ordering the test, patients knowing that the test is needed and taking the initiative to have the test done, and the results being communicated to the healthcare practitioner who is managing the patient's diabetes. These are considered primary drivers which are either achieved together or addressed as targets towards achieving the

Table 32.1 Project management and improvement tools

Tool	Purpose	Elements	Product
Driver diagram When: Step 2	Visual representation of an aim and the factors and activities that impact the aim	Aim: Primary factors – need to be influenced to achieve the aim Secondary factors – activities that impact the primary factors	Theory of change
Fishbone diagram When: Step 2	Outline of the factors that influence an outcome	Branches may include people, processes, policy, methods, materials and environmental factors	Hypothesis of causes of a problem
Gantt chart When: Step 3	Illustration of a schedule for project completion	Project milestones and elements, time and status	Progress made towards an aim
Process flowchart When: Step 3	Visual representation of a process and the people involved	Symbols used to depict start and end, steps in the process and decision points	Pictorial representation of a process
Plan–do–study–act (PDSA) When: Steps 2–6	Model for Improvement intended to test change by planning it, trying it, observing the results and acting on what is learned	**Plan** – the test or observation, including a plan for collecting data **Do** – try out the test on a small scale **Study** – set aside time to analyse the data and study the results **Act** – refine the change, based on what was learned from the test	Knowledge about whether a strategy led to improvement

Purpose
• Guide implementation of a change

Characteristics
• Three or more levels that outline the
  1. Aim
  2. Factors that influence the aim
  3. Activities that act on factors

It looks like:

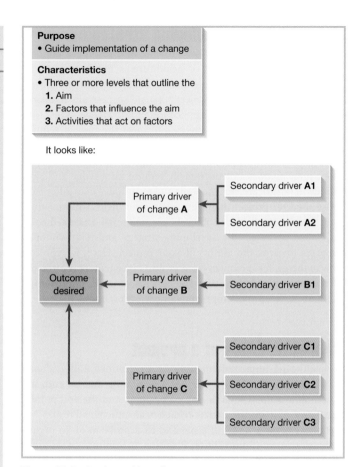

Figure 32.2 Putting a driver diagram to use

of the need for an A1c test, and communication of test results (Figure 32.3). The 'people' involved in the process may include practitioners, administrative staff, lab personnel and the patients. The 'systems' involved would be related to communication between the practitioners and the patient, the patient and the lab where the

Purpose
• Explore possible causes of a problem

Characteristics
• Potential causes to consider – people, environment, materials, methods and equipment

It looks like:

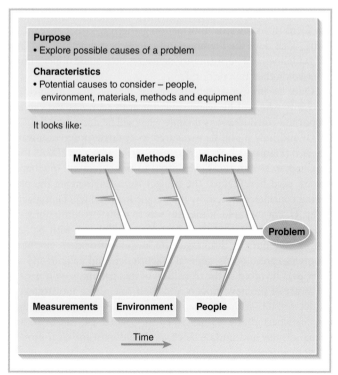

Figure 32.3 Putting a fishbone diagram to use

aim. The secondary drivers impact the primary drivers and may include ongoing monitoring of blood test results, access to a phlebotomy service and a process for sending results to practitioners. Each of the 'drivers' outlined as contributing towards the aim should be measurable so that the diagram provides a complete picture of a strategy for achieving an aim and how to measure progress.

If you are beginning with a problem or an 'effect' and your aim is to better understand the 'causes' to understand how to fix it, you could use a fishbone diagram. If the problem was incomplete diabetic A1c tests, you could think through the potential factors that are contributing to the tests not being completed. To categorise the potential causes, consider the methods, the people and the systems involved in completing an HbA1c test. There is no standard for categorising the potential causes, but some categories to consider include the 4 M's – methods, machines, materials and manpower; the 4 P's – place, procedure, people and policies; and the 4 S's – surroundings, suppliers, systems and skills. Some of the 'methods' we could explore relate to test ordering, patient awareness

A1c test is completed, and the lab and the practitioner. As you are identifying each of these factors, consider how each is contributing to the problem and why it is happening. Items that appear in more than one category can be considered most likely causes and can be further discussed and prioritised as contributing factors. The product of a fishbone diagram is a list of potential causes that can then be used to identify an improvement strategy.

A process flowchart can be useful at various points in your exploration of a problem or a solution, or in the management of a project through to completion. Figure 32.1 is a process flowchart that outlines how to execute a project plan. This tool outlines activities and sometimes decision points along a project cycle. For example, if we mapped out a plan for diabetes management, completing A1c tests before a practitioner visit would be one of the steps explored along the process from ordering the test to the practitioner receiving the results. This visual representation of a process can help identify each step and how to proceed at various decision points. The result is a mapped-out process and a plan for achieving your project aim(s), which help to maintain focus along the project cycle. See Chapters 26 and 36 for examples.

A Gantt chart can be used to monitor progress towards project aims. This tool, similar to a timeline, outlines project deliverables on the y-axis and time on the x-axis. A Gantt chart is useful for monitoring deliverables and communicating the status of a project. It complements a process flowchart when time is associated with each project element represented in the flowchart (Figure 32.4).

Both tools present project managers with a framework for organising elements of a project and a mechanism for communicating with the individuals engaged in the project.

Conclusion

Healthcare improvements must be achieved by leader managers – those dedicated to the organisation and its long-term success. Becoming a leader manager begins with recognising that, as a health professional, you have two jobs: job 1 is doing the work, which is providing healthcare; and job 2 is improving it. Armed with the knowledge of how to manage a project and the tools presented in this chapter, you can become a leader manager and be successful in job 2.

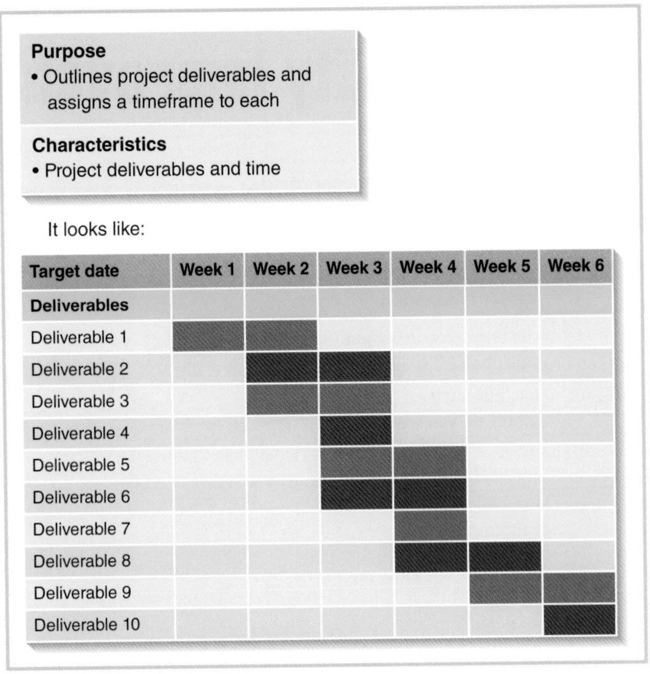

Purpose
• Outlines project deliverables and assigns a timeframe to each

Characteristics
• Project deliverables and time

It looks like:

Target date	Week 1	Week 2	Week 3	Week 4	Week 5	Week 6
Deliverables						
Deliverable 1	■	■				
Deliverable 2		■	■			
Deliverable 3		■				
Deliverable 4			■			
Deliverable 5			■	■		
Deliverable 6			■	■		
Deliverable 7				■		
Deliverable 8				■	■	
Deliverable 9					■	■
Deliverable 10						■

Figure 32.4 Putting a Gantt chart to use

33 Quality improvement in psychiatry

Figure 33.1 Plan–do–study–act (PDSA) cycles for increasing use of the Alcohol Use Disorders Identification Test – Consumption (AUDIT-C)

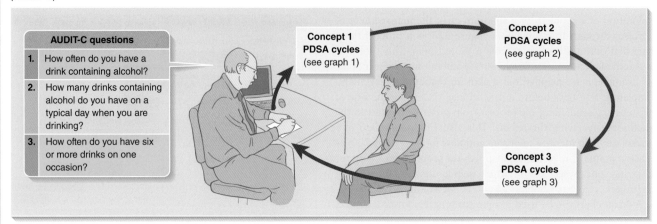

AUDIT-C questions

1. How often do you have a drink containing alcohol?
2. How many drinks containing alcohol do you have on a typical day when you are drinking?
3. How often do you have six or more drinks on one occasion?

Concept 1 PDSA cycles (see graph 1)

Concept 2 PDSA cycles (see graph 2)

Concept 3 PDSA cycles (see graph 3)

Figure 33.2 Root cause analysis on low rates of alcohol screening

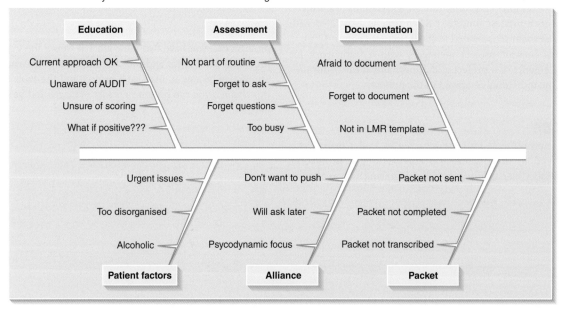

Education
- Current approach OK
- Unaware of AUDIT
- Unsure of scoring
- What if positive???

Assessment
- Not part of routine
- Forget to ask
- Forget questions
- Too busy

Documentation
- Afraid to document
- Forget to document
- Not in LMR template

Patient factors
- Urgent issues
- Too disorganised
- Alcoholic

Alliance
- Don't want to push
- Will ask later
- Psycodynamic focus

Packet
- Packet not sent
- Packet not completed
- Packet not transcribed

Figure 33.3 Control charts for monitoring improvement in the rate of Alcohol Use Disorders Identification Test – Consumption (AUDIT-C) utilisation

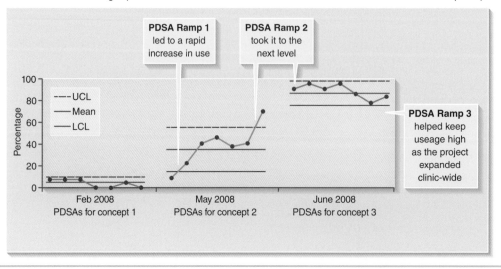

PDSA Ramp 1 led to a rapid increase in use

PDSA Ramp 2 took it to the next level

PDSA Ramp 3 helped keep useage high as the project expanded clinic-wide

- - - - UCL
——— Mean
——— LCL

Percentage

Feb 2008
PDSAs for concept 1

May 2008
PDSAs for concept 2

June 2008
PDSAs for concept 3

Patient Safety and Healthcare Improvement at a Glance, First Edition. Edited by Sukhmeet S. Panesar, Andrew Carson-Stevens, Sarah A. Salvilla and Aziz Sheikh
© 2014 John Wiley & Sons, Ltd. Published 2014 by John Wiley & Sons, Ltd.

Introduction

The nature of psychiatric disorders and their treatment present a unique set of challenges for quality improvement. Stigma about mental illness, a high degree of inter-provider variability in the approach to diagnosis and treatment, and a relative lack of objective tools for screening, diagnosis and outcome measurement are common challenges. The World Health Organization (WHO) estimates that harmful use of alcohol accounts for approximately 3.8% of all deaths (2.3 million) around the world, and studies show the mortality rate is increased threefold when alcohol use disorders are comorbid with mental illness. Despite these data, the use of validated alcohol use screening tools remains low in the majority of outpatient psychiatric clinics.

The aim in this example is to increase the use of a scientifically validated tool to screen for alcohol use disorder in a general psychiatry outpatient clinic. The goal was to increase use of the tool during new intake evaluations from 4% to 50%. Let's look at how the Model for Improvement was used to achieve this goal.

Strategy for change

Three key concepts that resulted in the biggest changes during the improvement project are outlined; the plan–do–study–act (PDSA) cycles that developed and tested the change ideas are summarised. The three concepts informed secondary drivers in a larger driver diagram.

Concept 1: Provide training and support for tool use – Education and 'cheat sheets' will increase the rate of use of a scientifically validated screening tool for alcohol use disorders.

Summary of plans made in PDSA cycles:

1 Create a team comprising department leadership, substance abuse specialists and frontline clinicians from the outpatient mental health clinic.

2 Use a fishbone template to identify potential causes of low rates of alcohol screening (see Figure 33.2).

3 Establish a baseline from previous patient notes in the past 3 months (see the control chart in Figure 33.3).

4 Expand fishbone categories through team discussion to include specific elements felt by the team to contribute to low rates of screening.

5 Identify a pilot group of mental health clinicians that agree to pilot a simple-to-use and scientifically valid screening tool (the Alcohol Use Disorders Identification Test – Consumption (AUDIT-C)). An educational session was convened; clinicians were provided with a 'cheat sheet' (a prompt with key details) to guide use of the tool during the initial assessment. Each clinician asked to trial the tool in their practice and provided feedback at a follow-up educational session.

Summary of learning from collected data and feedback from PDSAs run for Concept 1: Only 4% of charts showed evidence of use of a standardised screening instrument. In one month, the rate of screening usage increased to 40%, but the improvement plateaued, and towards the end of the month there was evidence of decreased usage. This prompted the team to determine why; the issues identified in the fishbone diagram combined with clinician feedback guided further tests in subsequent PDSA cycles.

Concept 2: Regular feedback to clinicians – Implementing an audit and feedback process to understand barriers to embedding the intervention will help sustain our gains.

Summary of plans made in PDSA cycles:

6 Schedule audit and feedback sessions with the pilot clinicians to explore why some clinicians were exhibiting more consistent uptake of the screening tool, while others appeared to lag behind, and to better understand their individual barriers. The sessions would reiterate the importance of tool use, present data on the uptake by other colleagues, and use the fishbone diagram to guide discussion to help recognise the multiple factors that may be prohibiting tool use.

Summary of learning from collected data and feedback from PDSAs run for Concept 2: One-to-one feedback and discussion with lagging clinicians comprised a more powerful method for improving uptake than group feedback sessions. Control charts were a consistent source of guidance to judge the impact of our feedback efforts and identify potential clinicians to target. Use increased from 40% to 90% in 4 months. New mean and upper control and lower control limits were created for the project. Consistent pushback from clinicians about financial compensation for completing these tools with patients was noted.

Concept 3: Financial incentives – Including the use of incentives will encourage other staff (not in the pilot group) to partake in education and use the tool during emergency psychiatric admissions.

Summary of plans made in PDSA cycles:

7 Determine whether the uptake of AUDIC-C can be increased through a targeted incentives programme. All clinicians were informed of the AUDIT-C project, and the benefits were identified by clinicians in the trial group. Details about the new incentives programme were included via email messages and announcements at department-wide meetings. Incentive payments were provided to clinicians who partook in education sessions and then used AUDIT-C in initial intakes.

Summary of learning from collected data and feedback from PDSAs run for Concept 3: The 93% screening target set by the US Veterans Administration was exceeded. Financial incentives advised by the trial group proved popular for wider uptake. Additional work was needed to improve the incentives programme and to embed AUDIT-C into electronic templates. Furthermore, a set of brief treatment algorithms was developed to support clinical decision making using the AUDIT-C scoring. The team felt that a continuous learning opportunity was generated from using the Model for Improvement to develop changes and test-specific change ideas based on the concepts underpinning key primary and secondary drivers in the driver diagram (see Chapter 34 for an example of a driver diagram).

34 Quality improvement in intensive care

Figure 34.1 A critical care driver diagram

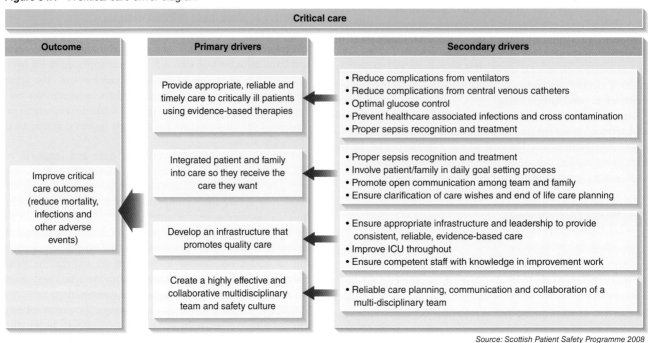

Source: Scottish Patient Safety Programme 2008

Figure 34.2 Intensive care unit average length of stay, (August 2007–August 2012)

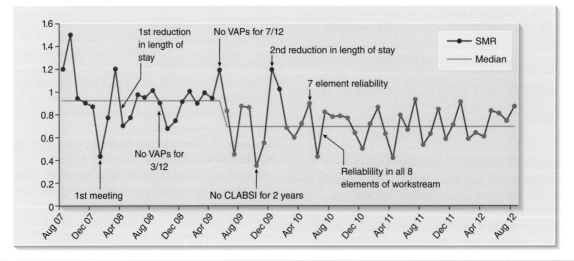

Patient Safety and Healthcare Improvement at a Glance, First Edition. Edited by Sukhmeet S. Panesar, Andrew Carson-Stevens, Sarah A. Salvilla and Aziz Sheikh
© 2014 John Wiley & Sons, Ltd. Published 2014 by John Wiley & Sons, Ltd.

Introduction

Patient safety is core to all aspects of intensive care training, education and standards. The strong history of nurturing a safety culture in the speciality, learning from error, preventing harm and working as part of a multi-disciplinary team all contribute to the disciplines of safety and critical care. Bundles, processes and checklists are all terms now familiar to those working in intensive care units (ICUs).

Problem

An audit in an ICU revealed the incidence of ventilator-associated pneumonia (VAP) to be 17 per 1000 ventilated days and the central line–associated bloodstream infection (CLABSI) rate to be 22 per 1000 catheter days. Improvement was needed in terms of reducing waste, harm and unwarranted variation within clinical practice and healthcare delivery.

A multi-disciplinary team was established that comprised medical and nursing staff, a pharmacist, a physiotherapist and a dietician. The team met regularly in person or through online discussion in order to problem-solve issues and guide testing of change.

Intervention

Following an initial brainstorming at a weekly multi-disciplinary team meeting, a critical care **driver diagram** (Figure 34.1) and a **Pareto chart** (Figure 34.3) were used to highlight the main challenges and consider how the change package could address these challenges. A Pareto chart is used to graphically summarise and display the relative importance of the differences between groups of data; the lengths of the bars represent frequency of the issues and are arranged in descending order to visually depict which situations are most significant. A driver diagram helped to clarify our understanding of how our own ICU system worked and identify the changes we thought were needed for improvement.

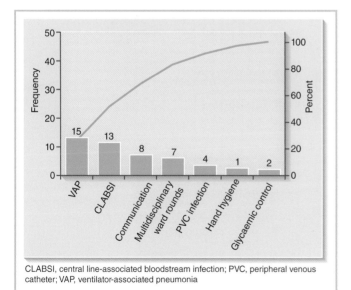

CLABSI, central line-associated bloodstream infection; PVC, peripheral venous catheter; VAP, ventilator-associated pneumonia

Figure 34.3 Pareto chart displaying ICU challenges

The aim of the project was to reduce ICU standardised mortality ratio by 10% between December 2007 and December 2012. The change package comprised eight key processes that could assist in delivering reliable critical care:

1 Ventilator-associated pneumonia bundle
2 Central venous catheter (CVC) insertion bundle
3 Central venous catheter maintenance
4 Peripheral venous catheter (PVC) maintenance
5 Multi-disciplinary ward rounds
6 Daily goals
7 Glycaemic control
8 Hand hygiene

Patient stories, both good and bad, were used to describe areas of good practice and establish a burning platform when suboptimal care had occurred (see Chapter 28). **Care bundles** to ensure good compliance with evidence-based practice as well as **checklists** for high-risk or complicated procedures (e.g. rapid sequence induction and intubation, and CVC insertion) were also used.

Change strategy and measurement

The **Model for Improvement** was used to initiate a continuous series of small-scale tests of change performed by a multi-disciplinary team. First it started small with one patient, one nurse and one doctor on one shift. Once some understanding about the process was gained and it was being delivered reliably, it was then tested with three, then five, patients, at different times of the day, prior to its rollout to the whole ICU.

Motivation and communication with members of the team were facilitated by twice-daily safety briefings and an open and transparent display of infection rates in the middle of the clinical area in the ICU. Real-time assessment of data was displayed on daily and monthly run charts.

Results

Significant reductions in VAP and CLABSI rates were achieved with more than 250 days and 730 days between events, respectively. This was associated with a 0.5 day reduction on time spent on a ventilator, as well as a 1.1 day reduction in ICU length of stay. The 5 **Whys** (see Chapter 27) were used to explore whether the reduction in length of stay could be explained by reasons other than a reduction in hospital-acquired infection rates (i.e. less sick patients). The analysis revealed that despite an increase in the complexity and severity of cases, the ICU average length of stay had still reduced by 1.1 days with a corresponding 0.23 reduction in the standardised mortality ratio from 0.92 to 0.69 (see the run chart in Figure 34.2).

Conclusions

The public display of the ICU's infection rates helped the ICU transition to a transparent and safety-focused culture. Multiple small-scale tests of change, guided by the Model for Improvement, were integral to changing practice in this high-risk environment. Bundles of care, daily goals and checklists also helped to produce high-quality, reliable healthcare.

35 Quality improvement in obstetrics

Figure 35.1 CTG score sticker

No:	Date:		Time:	
Define risk			High	
			Low	
C: 10		Temp:	Pulse:	
Feature	**0** Reassuring	**1** Non-reassuring	**2** Abnormal	
BRA Start = Now =	110–169	100–109 161–180 **Rising baseline**	<100 >180	
V	>5 bpm	<5 bpm for 40–90 min	<5 bpm for >90 mins Sinusoidal >10 mins	
A	Present	Absent*		
D	**None** **Typicals** <50% for <90 min	**Typicals** >50% contractions > 90 min **Brady** up to 3 min	**Atypicals** >50% contractions >30 min **Late** >30 min **Brady** >3 min	
O	0 = Normal	1 = Suspicious	≥2 = pathological	
Plan	Continue	Conservative, e.g. reposition, fluids, antipyretics, adjust synto	FBS Expedite delivery if FBS impossible or acute event, e.g. brady >3 mins	
Who	Case midwife	Snr midwife	Fresh eyes	Doctor
Name				
Sign				

Figure 35.2 The 4 S's sticker

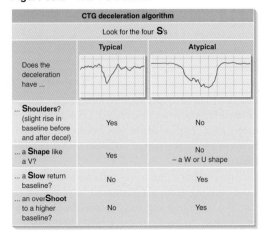

CTG deceleration algorithm		
Look for the four **S**'s		
	Typical	**Atypical**
Does the deceleration have ...		
... **Shoulders**? (slight rise in baseline before and after decel)	Yes	No
... a **Shape** like a V?	Yes	No – a W or U shape
... a **Slow** return baseline?	No	Yes
... an over**Shoot** to a higher baseline?	No	Yes

C = Contractions
BRA = Baseline rate
V = Variability
A = Accelerations
D = Decelerations
O = Overall Impression

Figure 35.3 Cardiotograph model of improvement

What are we trying to accomplish?

To redesign the current process of cardiotograph (CTG) interpretation to reduce the number of cases misclassified and resulting in morbidity

How will we know that a change is an improvement?

Goal	Measure	Type of measure
Decreased the number of cases of CTGs that are misclassified	% CTGs correctly classified	Outcome
Increased staff knowledge of National Institute for Health and Care Excellence (NICE) CTG classification criteria	Score of the pre-and post-test	Process
Increased staff compliance with the new process	% compliance to new process	Process
Increase midwife confidence	Midwife confidence score	Balancing

Figure 35.4 Percentage of cardiotographs (CTGs) misclassified on Ward 1 (p-chart)

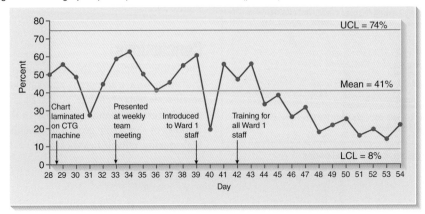

Patient Safety and Healthcare Improvement at a Glance, First Edition. Edited by Sukhmeet S. Panesar, Andrew Carson-Stevens, Sarah A. Salvilla and Aziz Sheikh
© 2014 John Wiley & Sons, Ltd. Published 2014 by John Wiley & Sons, Ltd.

Introduction

The cardiotograph (CTG) is a method of assessing foetal heart rate to identify babies at risk of complication (which can include death) as a result of the birthing process. The interpretation of CTGs was acknowledged to be poor at a large university teaching hospital, despite regular CTG training and the use of standardised stickers. An audit by a senior midwife showed deficiencies in classification (52%), inappropriate action (56%) and inadequate documentation (24%) of the CTGs of 25 women in November 2012. National medical malpractice claims supported a strong argument to make this a focus for a quality improvement project because mistakes in CTG interpretation can result in cerebral palsy, resulting in over £2 billion of medical negligence claims in the United Kingdom over a 10 year period.

Aim

Ninety per cent correct classification and appropriate management of the CTG.

Intervention

Introduce a CTG classification sticker that was developed and successfully implemented at another hospital.

Timeline of change

Days 1–4: The specialist registrar obstetrics doctor (SpR) shows senior colleagues and peers a prototype of the CTG sticker. Feedback is negative as they feel that there is already a sticker system in place and 'another piece of paper' would not be helpful.

Days 7–11: SpR undertakes a brief survey with 34 midwives and 16 doctors, and identifies several key reasons for CTG misclassification:

• The CTG terminology and accompanying guidelines kept changing and had too many features to remember in an acute situation
• Decelerations (a feature of the heart rate slowing down) were the most confusing feature to interpret (95%). Many (72%) were unfamiliar with the difference between typical and atypical decelerations despite training day interventions
• Two stickers were already in use. Neither helped with accurate classification or management
• Frequent need for a second opinion as unsure, and CTG was over-classified as suspicious or pathological

SpR presented a new sticker to staff and received unanimous positive feedback about the layout (aided easier classification), credibility (incorporated both classification systems) and usefulness (served as a reference and an educational tool, and also prompted appropriate communication and management). Suggestions were made to include a chart or algorithm on the CTG machine to help distinguish between atypical and typical decelerations.

Days 10–11: Findings presented to midwifery manager.

Day 14: Findings presented by manager at the midwifery senior management meeting. Need for new sticker accepted, and colour coding suggested. Mock-up of CTG deceleration algorithm drawn up.

Day 19: Patient safety manager liked the tools and presented them at the quarterly organisation-wide Clinical Improvement in Maternity meeting. Both rejected by neighbouring hospitals in the same group as 'another piece of paper'.

Day 23: Manager and supervisors felt a pilot should go ahead and agreed to implement it as a printed CTG sheet before committing to sticker production.

Testing in practice

Days 24–25: SpR tests tools with six midwives on labour ward to use with one patient each per 12-hour shift. Feedback at end of each day shows tools to be effective and easy to use, but deceleration chart could be simpler.

Day 26: SpR analysed findings, and CTG sticker text strengthened by minimising wording. Deceleration algorithm honed down to a simple-to-remember '4 S's' (see Figures 35.1 and 35.2).

Day 27: Tools were updated, and findings were presented to team.

Day 28: Midwifery manager and supervisor laminate deceleration chart and attach to all CTG machines on labour ward.

Day 33: Tools and findings presented by SpR and patient safety manager to obstetricians at weekly CTG meeting to raise awareness. Initially rejected as 'another piece of paper' by consultants. Accepted by trainees and students as valuable – they took copies and photographs on their telephones for their own personal reference. Evidence and rationale for tools recognised after demonstration of correct classification with CTG error cases brought to meeting. Participants agreed to expand the new system with a trial week for all staff on the labour ward.

Days 39–43: Staff introduced to pilot and use of tools at handover. Ongoing education with tools in the form of informal reviews during the ward rounds to eliminate gaps in teaching and utilisation. Feedback and suggestions for improvement gathered daily.

Days 44–continuing: Project ongoing and continuing to build momentum and popularity with midwives and junior obstetric doctors.

Measures of improvement

Figure 35.3 outlines the process, outcome and balancing measures used during the improvement project. Run charts were made for each process and outcome measure.

Effects of change

Process measures improved in a short time. Staff adapted to the change. CTG stickers are now present on every machine in every room on the labour ward. Senior doctors and midwives have supported the project and have assigned a junior doctor to undertake a weekly analysis of 25 sets of notes to inform a run chart presented at the CTG meeting each week. Incorrectly analysed CTGs are used for teaching purposes.

Figure 35.4 is a control chart to display the percentage of CTGs misclassified on one of the participating wards in the improvement project. The Ward 1 team felt strongly that no CTGs should be misclassified if the rules within the tool were replied reliably; thus, they decided to chart the percentage of misclassifications, in which an overall downward trend was positive. Note that the team has annotated key project events on their chart. Can you identify special-cause rules 2, 5 and 6 (see Chapter 24 for a recap) in Figure 35.4?

Learning for others

Redesign of an existing tool can encourage buy-in and acceptance, and can be cost-effective, especially if stakeholders with authority are involved early on to ensure leverage and sustainability.

36 Quality improvement in surgery

Figure 36.1 OR process improvement map

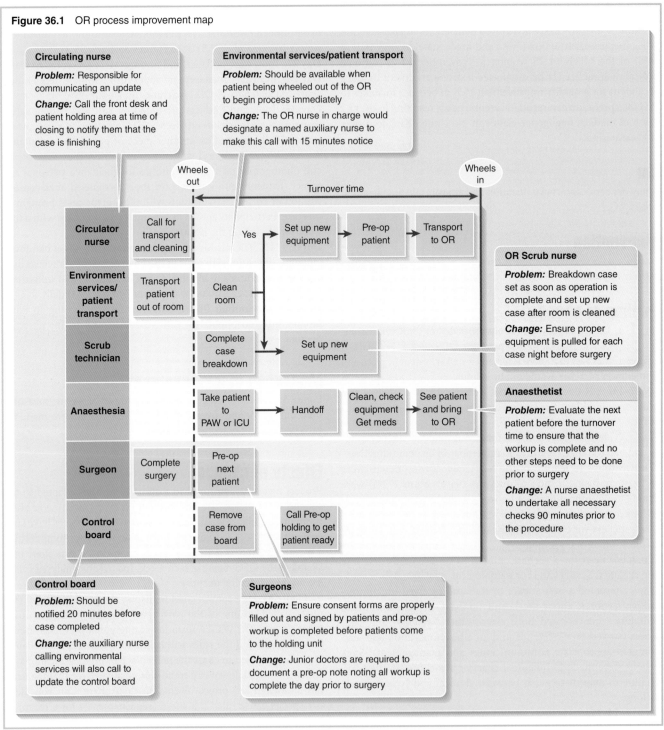

Circulating nurse

Problem: Responsible for communicating an update

Change: Call the front desk and patient holding area at time of closing to notify them that the case is finishing

Environmental services/patient transport

Problem: Should be available when patient being wheeled out of the OR to begin process immediately

Change: The OR nurse in charge would designate a named auxiliary nurse to make this call with 15 minutes notice

Wheels out

Wheels in

Turnover time

Circulator nurse	Call for transport and cleaning	Yes →	Set up new equipment	Pre-op patient	Transport to OR
Environment services/ patient transport	Transport patient out of room	Clean room			
Scrub technician		Complete case breakdown	Set up new equipment		
Anaesthesia		Take patient to PAW or ICU	Handoff	Clean, check equipment Get meds	See patient and bring to OR
Surgeon	Complete surgery	Pre-op next patient			
Control board		Remove case from board	Call Pre-op holding to get patient ready		

OR Scrub nurse

Problem: Breakdown case set as soon as operation is complete and set up new case after room is cleaned

Change: Ensure proper equipment is pulled for each case night before surgery

Anaesthetist

Problem: Evaluate the next patient before the turnover time to ensure that the workup is complete and no other steps need to be done prior to surgery

Change: A nurse anaesthetist to undertake all necessary checks 90 minutes prior to the procedure

Control board

Problem: Should be notified 20 minutes before case completed

Change: the auxiliary nurse calling environmental services will also call to update the control board

Surgeons

Problem: Ensure consent forms are properly filled out and signed by patients and pre-op workup is completed before patients come to the holding unit

Change: Junior doctors are required to document a pre-op note noting all workup is complete the day prior to surgery

Patient Safety and Healthcare Improvement at a Glance, First Edition. Edited by Sukhmeet S. Panesar, Andrew Carson-Stevens, Sarah A. Salvilla and Aziz Sheikh
© 2014 John Wiley & Sons, Ltd. Published 2014 by John Wiley & Sons, Ltd.

Problem

Operating room (OR) turnover time can be a cause of inefficiency in surgery. This has many implications, including delays in scheduled operations, staff overtime costs and patient and healthcare professional dissatisfaction.

A busy surgical department in a large US teaching hospital wanted to improve the quality of the operative experience for surgical patients. When the process was audited, turnover times were noted as double the national average. A multi-disciplinary team approach was initiated to engage all stakeholders in a process-mapping exercise to better understand the current system and determine why the process was failing. Insights from this learning process were used to redesign existing processes.

Experience of running a process-mapping activity

A process-interaction map shows steps performed at key interactions between functions (inputs and outputs) and activities (actions to move the process along that are often performed in parallel). This allows team members to understand areas of waste and redundancy and find 'hot spot' areas to focus improvement efforts.

Step 1: Define the problem

This was defined as: 'To reduce OR turnover time (the time between a patient leaving and another patient being brought in as the next case) by 50%'.

Step 2: Establishing the team

The OR turnover process requires a team effort, involving surgeons, anaesthetists, scrub nurses, auxiliary nursing staff, porters and ward nurses. Having key opinion leaders from each group was vital for project credibility. Bringing multiple professionals to the table resulted in some disagreement about the perceived processes – each member of the team had a unique view of the system and valued processes differently. When one group was not represented, it was difficult to raise questions about their contributions since the answers were not in the room (e.g. who schedules the porters? And who communicates with them if there is a delay?).

A neutral facilitator oversaw the process-mapping activity, helped to focus attention on the problems being discussed, prevented meetings from running off target and kept the group on track to accomplish the goals initially agreed at the outset.

Step 3: Mapping the 'as is' process

A process map was constructed to visually depict the way the OR was currently being run. A large-scale image of the process was drawn, and small, coloured sticky notes were added to highlight value-adding and non-value-adding activities.

The sticky notes focused on problem areas that required attention and decision making. Each step was outlined in terms of who was involved, inputs and outputs, and an estimate of the time it took for each step.

Step 4: Establish measures for improvement and propose changes

The next goal was to find measurable changes for each group to help improve the system. In Figure 36.1, each key professional role was identified with their respective responsibilities during the turnover time highlighted. Problem areas involving each group were identified, and the team proposed agreeable changes collectively.

Step 5: Mapping the 'should be' process and implementation

Once improvements and changes had been identified and agreed upon by the group, a 'should be' map was created. A pilot was launched in one operating room. A named team member was responsible for documenting the times for each process during each turnover. A team debriefing occurred every day after the second turnover to discuss what went right and wrong during the turnovers and the challenges that the team faced. Frequent plan–do–study–act (PDSA) cycles brought light to individual processes that required some adjustment.

Changes guided by the process map

By the end of the first day, the turnover time had been reduced by 50%, in keeping with acceptable national standards. The team immediately realised that a major reason for change was the improvement in communication between the teams and individual ownership of the steps taken by each team member in the process flow. In order to sustain the change, factors that resulted in reverting back to the old processes (i.e. staff who missed the initial trial period continued to use the old method) were identified using a fishbone diagram. The Model for Improvement was used to test change ideas to mitigate the impact of those factors. A run chart of turnover time is now kept on display in the OR to ensure that the turnover time remains at a time deemed reasonable by team members.

37 Population health and improvement

Figure 37.1 A population health view of cardiovascular disease (CVD): socio-economic contributory factors, physical consequences and financial burden

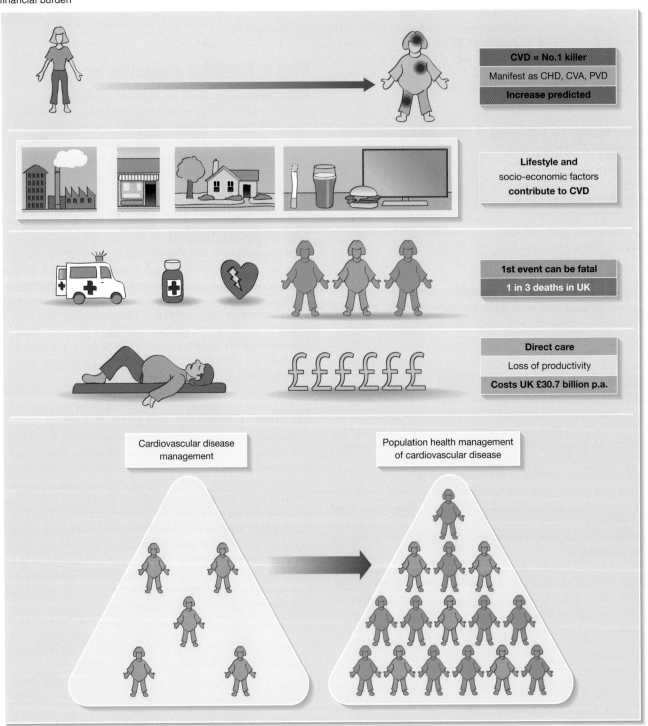

Patient Safety and Healthcare Improvement at a Glance, First Edition. Edited by Sukhmeet S. Panesar, Andrew Carson-Stevens, Sarah A. Salvilla and Aziz Sheikh
© 2014 John Wiley & Sons, Ltd. Published 2014 by John Wiley & Sons, Ltd.

Introduction

Looking beyond the smaller-scale improvement considered so far, here we will consider how visions of quality care are delivered to an entire population. 'Population health', similar to public health, explores factors that determine health and disease in populations and also works to develop and evaluate the impact of interventions to improve the health and wellbeing of the public. To think at a population level, a group of patients who share a common risk factor, health goal or condition need to be defined. Then, the health outcomes of the patient population can be considered, the health determinants that influence them can be identified and the policies and interventions that impact those determinants can be brought together to best understand and develop improvement ideas for potential targets to improve health outcomes. This strategy relies on access to information about a variety of factors that influence health, as well as a willingness of healthcare stakeholders at all levels to put the information to use in order to devise an approach to result in sustainable improvements for patient populations.

Prevention of cardiovascular disease

The World Health Organization (WHO) preventive strategy for reducing cardiovascular disease (CVD) focused on a population-based approach for managing people at high risk of either developing or worsening already-established CVD. To tackle mass disease, reducing risk factor levels in those at highest risk either without CVD or with established CVD is achieved by targeting medical risk factors and unhealthy lifestyle behaviours. For example, given the causal relationship between salt intake and blood pressure, reducing dietary sodium intake could be beneficial. WHO estimates that 49% of all coronary heart disease (CHD) and 62% of all strokes are attributable to high blood pressure. In most Western countries, the habitual salt intake is about 10 g a day – twice the level recommended by WHO. Thus, it is predicted in the United States that a 3 g dietary salt reduction per day would reduce the annual number of new cases of CHD by 60,000, stroke by 32,000 and myocardial infarction by 54,000 and the number of deaths from any cause by 44,000. A population-based approach requires prevention to be focused on groups, rather than individuals, such as those with CVD or those without, or those with a particular risk factor or those without. Research studies have demonstrated that it is possible to see up to 50% reductions in CVD mortality due to changes in risk factors, with 40% due to improvements in treatments.

Barriers to implementation

To successfully achieve this larger scale thinking, buy-in at the clinical level is essential. However, there can be barriers to implementing CVD prevention guidelines, including time constraints, a sense that preventive strategies are not effective, confusion over which risk assessment tool to use, inadequate training and the potential for adverse influences on clinician–patient relationships.

A large UK study (ASPIRE-2-PREVENT) showed that there was a wide gap in the implementation of evidence-based medicine in vascular management in both hospital and primary care.

Amongst asymptomatic high-risk people, there was a large proportion not achieving lifestyle, risk factor level and therapeutic targets. Where guidelines are adhered to, the risk factor and therapeutic targets may be different to what the evidence base regards as optimum. For example, in the United Kingdom, a reason for not reaching the blood pressure and lipid targets in high-risk patients could be because general practitioners use the Quality Outcomes Framework audit targets of blood pressure of <150/90 mm Hg and a total cholesterol target of <5.0 mmol/l, which is higher than the optimal therapeutic targets of <140/80 mm Hg and <4.0 mmol/l advised by research respectively.

A large survey conducted by the British Heart Foundation, a UK charity, found that a third of people with high cholesterol and a quarter with high blood pressure do not take their medication correctly. This may be due to side effects and poor information about the benefits. Traditional advice giving can create resistance to change among patients. Merely telling someone they are at risk of developing a disease is rarely sufficient to change behaviour. Theories about behaviour change and research associated with them have clarified the need to look beyond approaches that are based simply upon delivering expert opinions. Patients prefer a more patient-centred approach to consultations rather than more directive advice giving, for example a nurse-co-ordinated multi-disciplinary prevention programme for high-risk individuals and those with CVD in hospitals and primary care practices. The approach of eight visits over a 16-week programme, involving dieticians, physical activity specialists and cardiologists, led to healthier diet, improved physical activity and more effective control of blood pressure for patients and their partners in eight European countries.

Opportunities to reduce CVD require population-based strategies including legislative changes to help reduce, for example, smoking, trans fat consumption and dietary sodium consumption. The United Kingdom, Portugal, Finland and Japan have reduced population-wide salt intake through a combination of regulations on the salt content in processed foods, food labelling and public education. Legislative changes to increase the facilities and opportunities for exercise can further augment the population-based preventive approach.

Conclusion

Tackling the burden of preventative disease is an important clinical and societal goal. Healthcare professionals can play a big role in disease prevention since many patients remain undiagnosed and untreated, and there are treatment gaps even among patients with established disease. Barriers to population-based efforts are candidate areas for improvement projects locally (e.g. in general practice, or prior to patient discharge in hospitals). The improvement methods and tools in Chapters 21–36 can be used to develop improvement initiatives that focus on disease prevention (e.g. promoting better cardiovascular health to South Asian men) and health promotion (e.g. healthcare student-led projects to promote healthy eating choices to primary school children). The Model for Improvement could be used to learn how to successfully adopt evidence-based interventions into clinical practice.

Further reading

Chapter 1: Basics of patient safety

- Baker GR, Norton PG, Flintoft V, Blais R, Brown A, Cox J, *et al.* The Canadian adverse events study: the incidence of adverse events among hospital patients in Canada. *CMAJ* 2004;170:1678–86.
- Brennan TA, Leape LL, Laird NM, Hebert L, Localio AR, Lawthers AG, *et al.* Incidence of adverse events and negligence in hospitalised patients: results of the Harvard Medical Practice Study I. 1991. *Qual Saf Health Care* 2004;13:145–51.
- Cooper JB, Newbower RS, Long CD, McPeek B. Preventable anesthesia mishaps: a study of human factors. *Anesthesiology.* 1978;49(6):399–406
- Davis P, Lay-Yee R, Briant R, Ali W, Scott A, Schug S. Adverse events in New Zealand public hospitals. I. Occurrence and impact. *N Z Med J* 2002;115:U271.
- Department of Health. *An Organisation With a Memory.* London: Stationery Office, 2000. Available at: http://webarchive.nationalarchives.gov.uk/+/www.dh.gov.uk/en/AboutUs/MinistersAndDepartmentLeaders/ChiefMedicalOfficer/ProgressOnPolicy/ProgressBrowsableDocument/DH_5016613 (accessed 5 November 2013).
- de Vries EN, Ramrattan MA, Smorenburg SM, Gouma DJ, Boermeester MA. The incidence and nature of in-hospital adverse events: a systematic review. *Qual Saf Health Care.* 2008;17(3):216–223.
- Hogan H, Healey F, Neale G, Thomson R, Vincent C, Black N. Preventable deaths due to problems in care in English acute hospitals: a retrospective case record review study. *BMJ Qual Saf.* 2012;21(9):737–45.
- Institute of Medicine (IOM). *Crossing the Quality Chasm.* Washington, DC: National Academy Press, 2001. Available at: http://www.iom.edu/Global/News%20Announcements/Crossing-the-Quality-Chasm-The-IOM-Health-Care-Quality-Initiative.aspx (accessed 5 November 2013).
- Institute of Medicine (IOM). *To Err Is Human: Building a Safer Health System.* Washington, DC: National Academies Press, 2000.
- Rasmussen J. Skills, rules and knowledge; signals, signs and symbols, and other distinctions in human performance models. *IEEE Trans Sys, Man, Cyber* 1983;13(3):257–66.
- Reason J. Human error: models and management. *BMJ* 2000;320(7237):768–70.
- Runciman W, Hibbert P, Thomson R, Van Der Schaaf T, Sherman H, Lewalle P. Towards an international classification for patient safety: key concepts and terms. *Int J Qual Health Care* 2009;21(1):18–26.
- Schioler T, Lipczak H, Pedersen BL, Mogensen TS, Bech KB, Stockmarr A, *et al.* Incidence of adverse events in hospitals: a retrospective study of medical records. *Ugeskr Laeger* 2001;163:5370–8.
- Thomas EJ, Studdert DM, Burstin HR, Orav EJ, Zeena T, Williams EJ, *et al.* Incidence and types of adverse events and negligent care in Utah and Colorado. *Med Care* 2000;38:261–71.
- Vincent C, Neale G, Woloshynowych M. Adverse events in British hospitals: preliminary retrospective record review. *BMJ* 2001;322:517–9.
- Wilson RM, Runciman WB, Gibberd RW, Harrison BT, Newby L, Hamilton JD. The Quality in Australian Health Care study. *Med J Aust* 1995;163(9):458–71.
- World Health Organization. *WHO Patient Safety Curriculum Guide.* Topic 1. 2001. Available at: http://www.who.int/patientsafety/education/curriculum/who_mc_topic-1.pdf (accessed 5 November 2013).

Chapter 2: Understanding systems

- Department of Health. *An Organisation with a Memory.* London: Stationery Office, 2000. Available at: http://webarchive.nationalarchives.gov.uk/+/www.dh.gov.uk/en/AboutUs/MinistersAndDepartmentLeaders/ChiefMedicalOfficer/ProgressOnPolicy/ProgressBrowsableDocument/DH_5016613 (accessed 5 November 2013).
- Donabedian A. The quality of care: how can it be assessed? *JAMA* 1988;260:1743–8.
- Nolan T, Resar R, Haraden C, Griffin FA. *Improving the Reliability of Health Care.* IHI Innovation Series white paper. Cambridge, MA: Institute for Healthcare Improvement; 2004. Available at: http://www.ihi.org/knowledge/Pages/IHIWhitePapers/ImprovingtheReliabilityofHealthCare.aspx (accessed 31 December 2013).
- Reason, J. *Managing the Risks of Organizational Accidents.* Aldershot: Ashgate, 1997.
- The Health Foundation. How safe are clinical systems? Primary research into the reliability of systems within seven NHS organisations. The Health Foundation, 2011. Available at: http://www.health.org.uk/public/cms/75/76/313/587/How%20safe%20are%20clinical%20systems%20full%20length%20publication.pdf?realName=OaJgi3.pdf (accessed 1 May 2014)

Chapter 3: Quality and safety

- Berwick DM, Nolan TW, Whittington J. The triple aim: care, health, and cost. *Health Aff (Millwood)* 2008;27(3):759–69.
- Clinical microsystems. Available at: http://www.clinicalmicrosystem.org (accessed 31 December 2013).
- Donabedian A. Evaluating the quality of medical care. 1966. *Milbank Q* 2005;83(4):691–729.
- Institute for Healthcare Improvement (IHI) Triple aim initiative. Available at: http://www.ihi.org/offerings/Initiatives/TripleAIM/Pages/default.aspx (accessed 31 December 2013).
- Langley G, Moen R, Nolan K, Nolan T, Norman C, Provost L. *The Improvement Guide: A Practical Approach to Enhancing Organizational Performance,* 2nd ed. San Francisco: Jossey-Bass, 2009.
- Mitchell PH. Defining patient safety and quality care. In: Hughes RG, ed. *Patient Safety and Quality: An Evidence-Based Handbook for Nurses.* Rockville, MD: Agency for Healthcare Research and Quality, 2008. Available at: http://www.ncbi.nlm.nih.gov/books/NBK2681/ (accessed 5 November 2013).

Chapter 4: Human factors

- Carayon P, Schoofs Hundt A, Karsh B-T, Gurses AP, Alvarado CJ, Smith M, Flatley Brennan P. Work system design for patient safety:

Patient Safety and Healthcare Improvement at a Glance, First Edition. Edited by Sukhmeet S. Panesar, Andrew Carson-Stevens, Sarah A. Salvilla and Aziz Sheikh
© 2014 John Wiley & Sons, Ltd. Published 2014 by John Wiley & Sons, Ltd.

the SEIPS model. *Qual Saf Health Care* 2006;15:i50–8. doi:10.1136/qshc.2005.015842

• Carthey J. Implementing human factors in healthcare: taking further steps. Available at: http://www.chfg.org/wp-content/uploads/2013/05/Implementing-human-factors-in-healthcare-How-to-guide-volume-2-FINAL-2013_05_16.pdf (accessed 31 December 2013).

• Catchpole K. Defining clinical human factors. Available at: http://chfg.org/definition/defining-clinical-human-factors (accessed 31 December 2013).

• Patient Safety First. *Implementing Human Factors in Healthcare*. Available at: http://www.patientsafetyfirst.nhs.uk/ashx/Asset.ashx?path=/Intervention-support/Human%20Factors%20How-to%20Guide%20v1.2.pdf (accessed 5 November 2013).

• World Health Organization. Human factors. Available at: http://www.who.int/patientsafety/research/methods_measures/human_factors/en/ (accessed 5 November 2013).

Chapter 5: Teamwork and communication

• Canadian Patient Safety Institute. Canadian Framework for Teamwork and Communication. Available at: http://www.patientsafetyinstitute.ca/English/toolsResources/teamworkCommunication/Pages/default.aspx (accessed 5 November 2013).

• Health Foundation. Teamwork and communication. Available at: http://patientsafety.health.org.uk/area-of-care/safety-management/teamwork-and-communication (accessed 5 November 2013).

• Joint Commission on Accreditation of Healthcare Organizations. *The Joint Commission Guide to Improving Staff Communication*. Oakbrook Terrace, IL: Joint Commission Resources, 2005.

• Salas E, Cooke NJ, Rosen MA. On teams, teamwork, and team performance: discoveries and developments. *Hum Factors* 2008;50(3):540–7.

Chapter 6: Reporting and learning from errors

• Barach P, SD. Reporting and preventing medical mishaps: lessons from non-medical near miss reporting systems. *BMJ* 2000; 320: 759–63.

• Kingston MJ, Evans SM, Smith BJ, Berry JG. Attitudes of doctors and nurses towards incident reporting. *Med Journal of Australia* 2004; 181(5): 36–9.

• Lamont T, Scarpello J. National Patient Safety Agency: combining stories with statistics to minimise harm. *BMJ* 2009;339:b4489, doi: 10.1136/bmj.b4489

• Runciman WB, Edmonds MJ, Pradhan M. Setting priorities for patient safety. *Qual Saf Health Care* 2002; 11: 224–229.

• Sari A B-A, Sheldon TA, Cracknell A, Turnbull A. Sensitivity of routine system for reporting patient safety incidents in an NHS hospital: retrospective patient case note review. BMJ 2007;334: 79–83

• Vincent C. Incident reporting and patient safety. *BMJ* 2007; 334: 51.

• Woloshynowych M, Rogers S, Taylor-Adams S, Vincent C. The investigation and analysis of critical incidents and adverse events in healthcare. *Health Technology Assessment* 2005; 9(19): 1–143, iii.

• World Alliance for Patient Safety (2005). WHO Draft guidelines for adverse event reporting and learning systems. *WHO*, 2005

Chapter 7: Research in patient safety

• Herzer KR, Pronovost PJ. Motivating physicians to improve quality: light the intrinsic fire. *Am J Med Qual* 2013 Nov 18. [Epub ahead of print]

• Pronovost PJ, Goeschel CA, Marsteller JA, Sexton JB, Pham JC, Berenholtz SM. Framework for patient safety research and improvement. *Circulation* 2009;119(2):330–7.

• Pronovost PJ, Wachter RM. Progress in patient safety: a glass fuller than it seems. *Am J Med Qual* 2013 Aug 12. [Epub ahead of print]

• Romig M, Goeschel C, Pronovost P, Berenholtz SM. Integrating CUSP and TRIP to improve patient safety. *Hosp Pract (1995)* 2010;38(4):114–21.

• Selberg J, Pronovost P, Kaplan G. Culture conscious: leaders talk quality, change needed for improvement at virtual conference. *Mod Healthcare* 2013;43(24):18, 22.

• Shekelle PG, Pronovost PJ, Wachter RM, *et al.* Advancing the science of patient safety. *Ann Intern Med* 2011;154(10):693–6.

• Wachter RM, Pronovost P, Shekelle P. Strategies to improve patient safety: the evidence base matures. *Ann Intern Med* 2013 Mar 5;158(5 Pt 1):350–2.

• World Health Organization. *WHO Patient Safety Curriculum Guide. Topic 1.* 2001. Available at: http://www.who.int/patientsafety/education/curriculum/who_mc_topic-1.pdf (accessed 5 November 2013).

Chapter 8: Risk-based patient safety metrics

• Dr Foster Health. Available at: http://www.drfosterhealth.co.uk/ (accessed 5 November 2013).

• Institute of Medicine (IOM). *To Err Is Human: Building a Safer Health System.* Washington, DC: National Academies Press, 2000.

• Kmietowicz Z. Individual hospital data on 'never events' to be published every quarter. *BMJ* 2013;347:f7479.

• The Leapfrog Group. Available at: http://www.leapfroggroup.org/ (accessed 5 November 2013).

• Lilford R, Pronovost P. Using hospital mortality rates to judge hospital performance: a bad idea that just won't go away. *BMJ* 2010;340:c2016. Available at: http://www.bmj.com/content/340/bmj.c2016 (accessed 5 November 2013).

Chapter 9: Root cause analysis

• Institute for Healthcare Improvement (IHI). Cause and effect diagram. Available at: http://www.ihi.org/knowledge/Pages/Tools/CauseandEffectDiagram.aspx (accessed 31st December 2013).

• National Patient Safety Agency. Root cause analysis investigations. Available at: http://www.nrls.npsa.nhs.uk/resources/collections/root-cause-analysis/ (accessed 5 November 2013).

• Woloshynowych M, Rogers S, Taylor-Adams S, Vincent C. The investigation and analysis of critical incidents and adverse events in healthcare. *Health Technol Assess* 2005;9(19):1–143.

Chapter 10: Measuring safety culture

• Hansen LO, Williams MV, Singer SJ. Perceptions of hospital safety climate and incidence of readmission. *Health Services Research* 2011; 46(2):596–616.

• Haynes AB, Weiser TG, Berry WR, Lipsitz SR, Breizat AH, Dellinger EP, Dziekan G, Herbosa T, Kibatala PL, Lapitan MC, Merry AF, Reznick RK, Taylor B, Vats A, Gawande AA. Changes in safety attitude and relationship to decreased postoperative morbidity and mortality following implementation of a checklist-based surgical safety intervention. *BMJ Qual Saf* 2011;20(1):102–7.

• Health Foundation. Does improving safety culture affect patient safety outcomes? Available at: http://www.health.org.uk/public/cms/75/76/313/3078/Does%20improving%20safety%20culture%20affect%20outcomes.pdf?realName=fsu8Va.pdf (accessed 31 December 2013).

• Health Foundation. The importance of culture in patient safety. Available at: http://www.health.org.uk/news-and-events/newsletter/the-importance-of-culture-in-patient-safety (accessed 5 November 2013).

• Huang DT, Clermont G, Kong L, Weissfeld LA, Sexton JB, Rowan KM, Angus DC. Intensive care unit safety culture and outcomes: a US multicenter study. *Int J Qual Health Care* 2010; 22(3):151–61.

Chapter 11: Medication errors

• Bates DW. Using information technology to reduce rates of medication errors in hospitals. *BMJ* 2000 Mar 18;320(7237):788–91.

• Cousins DH, Gerrett D, Warner B. A review of medication incidents reported to the National Reporting and Learning System in England and Wales over 6 years (2005–2010). *Br J Clin Pharmacol* 2012;74(4):597–604.

• General Medical Council. GP prescribing errors research. 2012. Available at: http://www.gmc-uk.org/education/education_news/13037.asp (accessed 5 November 2013).

• Institute of Medicine (IOM). *Preventing Medication Errors.* Washington, DC: National Academies Press, 2007. Available at: http://books.nap.edu/openbook.php?record_id=11623 (accessed 31 December 2013).

• Noble DJ, Donaldson LJ. The quest to eliminate intrathecal vincristine errors: a 40-year journey. *Qual Saf Health Care* 2010;19(4):323–6.

Chapter 12: Surgical errors

• Amalberti R, Auroy Y, Berwick D, Barach P. Five system barriers to achieving ultrasafe health care. *Ann Intern Med* 2005;142(9):756–64.

• CTC Aviation Group. Non-technical skills. Available at: http://www.ctcaviation.com/airlines/aircrew_training/non_technical_skills (accessed 31 December 2013).

• Haynes AB, Weiser TG, Berry WR, Lipsitz SR, Breizat AH, Dellinger EP, Herbosa T, Joseph S, Kibatala PL, Lapitan MC, Merry AF, Moorthy K, Reznick RK, Taylor B, Gawande AA. Safe surgery saves lives study group: a surgical safety checklist to reduce morbidity and mortality in a global population. *N Engl J Med* 2009;360(5):491–9.

• National Patient Safety Agency. Surgical safety can be improved through better understanding of incidents. 2009. Available at: http://www.nrls.npsa.nhs.uk/resources/?entryid45=63054 (accessed 5 November 2013).

• Semel ME, Resch S, Haynes AB, Funk LM, Bader A, Berry WR, Weiser TG. Adopting a surgical safety checklist could save money and improve the quality of care in U.S. hospitals. *Health Aff (Millwood)* 2010;9:1593–9.

• Weiser TG, Regenbogen SE, Thompson KD, Haynes AB, Lipsitz SR, Berry WR, Gawande AA. An estimation of the global volume of surgery: a modelling strategy based on available data. *Lancet* 2008;372(9633):139–44.

Chapter 13: Diagnostic errors

• Croskerry P. Clinical cognition and diagnostic error: applications of a dual process model of reasoning. *Adv Health Sci Educ Theory Pract* 2009;14(Suppl 1):27–35.

• Graber ML, Kissam S, Payne VL, *et al.* Cognitive interventions to reduce diagnostic error: A narrative review. *BMJ Quality & Safety* 2012; 21(7), 535–57. doi: 10.1136/bmjqs-2011-000149

• Leape LL, Brennan TA, Laird N, Lawthers AG, Localio AR, Barnes BA, Hebert L, Newhouse JP, Weiler PC, Hiatt H. The nature of adverse events in hospitalized patients. Results of the Harvard Medical Practice Study II. *N Engl J Med* 1991;324(6):377–84.

• Newman-Toker DE, Pronovost PJ. Diagnostic errors: the next frontier for patient safety. *JAMA* 2009;301:1060–2.

• Shojania KG, Burton EC, McDonald KM, Goldman L. Changes in rates of autopsy-detected diagnostic errors over time: a systematic review. *JAMA* 2003;289:2849–56.

• Singh H. Diagnostic errors: moving beyond 'no respect' and getting ready for prime time. *BMJ Qual Saf* 2013;22(10):789–92.

• Singh H, Graber ML, Kissam SM, Sorensen AV, Lenfestey NF, Tant EM, Henriksen K, LaBresh KA. System-related interventions to reduce diagnostic errors: a narrative review. *BMJ Qual Saf* 2012;21(2):160–70.

• Singh H, Meyer AND, Thomas EJ. The frequency of diagnostic errors in outpatient care: Estimations from three large observational studies involving US adult populations. *BMJ Quality & Safety* 2014. doi:10.1136/bmjqs-2013-002627

Chapter 14: Maternal and child health errors

• Institute for Healthcare Improvement IHI). Perinatal improvement community. Available at http://www.ihi.org/offerings/MembershipsNetworks/collaboratives/PerinatalImprovementCommunity/Pages/default.aspx (accessed 31st December 2013).

• Prost A, Colbourn T, Seward N, et al. Women's groups practising participatory learning and action to improve maternal and newborn health in low-resource settings: a systematic review and meta-analysis. *Lancet* 2013; 381(9879):1736–46.

• Thaddeus S, Maine D. Too far to walk: maternal mortality in context. *Soc Sci Med* 1994;38:1091–110.

• World Health Organization. Launch of the WHO Safe Childbirth Checklist Collaboration. 2012. Available at: http://www.who.int/maternal_child_adolescent/news_events/news/2012/safe_childbirth_checklist/en/index.html (accessed 5 November 2013).

Chapter 15: Slips, trips and falls

• National Patient Safety Agency. Slips trips and falls data update. 2010. Available at: http://www.nrls.npsa.nhs.uk/resources/?entryid45=74567 (accessed 5 November 2013).

• National Institute for Health & Care Excellence. Clinical Guideline 109. Transient loss of consciousness in adults and young people NICE 2010. Available online at http://guidance.nice.org.uk/CG109

• National Institute for Health & Care Excellence Clinical Guideline 161 Falls: assessment and prevention of falls in older people NICE 2013. http://publications.nice.org.uk/falls-assessment-and-prevention-of-falls-in-older-people-cg161 (accessed 26 April 2014).

• Westby M, Davis S, Bullock I, et al. Transient loss of consciousness ("blackouts") management in adults and young people. London: National Clinical Guideline Centre for Acute and Chronic Conditions, Royal College of Physicians, 2010.

Chapter 16: Patient safety in paediatrics

• American Academy of Pediatrics. Principles of patient safety in pediatrics. *Pediatrics 2001*;107(6):1473–5. Available at: http://pediatrics.aappublications.org/content/107/6/1473.full (accessed 5 November 2013).

• Griffin FA, Resar RK. *IHI Global Trigger Tool for Measuring Adverse Events,* 2nd ed. IHI Innovation Series white paper. Cambridge, MA: Institute for Healthcare Improvement, 2009. Available at: http://www.ihi.org/knowledge/Pages/IHIWhitePapers/IHIGlobalTriggerToolWhitePaper.aspx (accessed 31 December 2013).

• Hollnagel E, Poulstrup A. [Patient safety in a new perspective]. *Ugeskr Laeger* 2012;174(45):2785–7.

- Lacey S, Smith JB, Cox K. Pediatric safety and quality. In: Hughes RG, ed. *Patient Safety and Quality: An Evidence-Based Handbook for Nurses*. Rockville, MD: Agency for Healthcare Research and Quality, 2008. Available at: http://www.ncbi.nlm.nih.gov/books/NBK2662/ (accessed 5 November 2013).
- National Institute for Health and Care Excellence (NICE). Feverish illness in children. Available at http://guidance.nice.org.uk/CG160 (accessed 31 December 2013).
- Nolan TW. System changes to improve patient safety. *BMJ* 2000;320(7237):771–3.
- Sutcliffe KM. High reliability organizations (HROs). *Best Pract Res Clin Anaesthesiol* 2011;25(2):133–44.
- Tibballs J, van der Jagt EW. Medical emergency and rapid response teams. *Pediatr Clin North Am* 2008;55(4):989–1010.
- Weick KE. Sense and reliability: a conversation with celebrated psychologist Karl E. Weick. Interview by Diane L. Coutu. *Harv Bus Rev* 2003;81(4):84–90, 123.
- Wennberg JE. Forty years of unwarranted variation – and still counting. *Health Pol* 2014;114(1):1–2.
- World Health Organization (WHO). 7 day mother baby mCheck tool. Available at: http://www.who.int/patientsafety/patients_for_patient/mother_baby/tool/en/index.html (accessed 31st December 2013).

Chapter 17: Technology in healthcare and e-iatrogenesis

- Avery AJ, Rodgers S, Cantrill JA, Armstrong S, Cresswell K, Eden M, Elliott RA, Howard R, Kendrick D, Morris CJ, Prescott RJ, Swanwick G, Franklin M, Putman K, Boyd M, Sheikh A. A pharmacist-led information technology intervention for medication errors (PINCER): a multicentre, cluster randomised, controlled trial and cost effectiveness analysis. *Lancet* 2012;379(9823):1310–9.
- McLean S, Sheikh A, Cresswell K, Nurmatov U, Mukherjee M, Hemmi A, Pagliari C. The impact of telehealthcare on the quality and safety of care: a systematic overview. *PLoS One* 2013;8(8):e71238.
- Oh H, Rizo C, Enkin M, Jadad A. What is e-health: a systematic review of published definitions. *J Med Internet Res* 2005;7(1):e1. Available at: http://www.ncbi.nlm.nih.gov/pmc/articles/PMC1550636/ (accessed 5 November 2013).

Chapter 18: Nosocomial infections

- Allegranzi B, Bagheri Nejad S, Combescure C, Graafmans W, Attar H, Donaldson L, Pittet D. Burden of endemic health-care-associated infection in developing countries: systematic review and meta-analysis. *Lancet* 2011;377(9761):228–41.
- Health Protection Agency. English National Point Prevalence Survey on Healthcare-associated Infections and Antimicrobial Use, 2011: preliminary data. 2011. Available at: http://www.hpa.org.uk/Topics/InfectiousDiseases/InfectionsAZ/HCAI/HCAIPointPrevalenceSurvey/ (accessed 5 November 2013).

Chapter 19: Mental health errors

- Appleby L, Shaw J, Kapur N, et al. Avoidable Deaths: Five year report of the National Confidential Inquiry into suicide and homicide by People with Mental Illness. Manchester: University of Manchester. 2006. Available from: http://www.medicine.manchester.ac.uk/psychiatry/research/suicide/prevention/nci/reports/ avoidabledeathsfullreport.pdf(accessed 17 April 2014).
- Department of Health. Refocusing the Care Programme Approach: Policy and Positive Practice Guidance. 2008. Available from: http://www.dh.gov.uk/en/Publicationsandstatistics/Publications/PublicationsPolicyAndGuidance/Dh_083647 (accessed 17 April 2014).
- General Medical Council. Confidentiality. Available from: http://www.gmc-uk.org/static/documents/content/Confidentiality_core_2009.pdf (accessed 17 April 2014).
- National Institute for Mental Health in England. Preventing Suicide: A Toolkit for Mental Health Services. 2003. Available from: http://kc.csip.org.uk/upload/SuicidePreventionToolkitweb.pdf (accessed 17 April 2014).
- National Mental Health Development Unit. Strategies to Reduce Missing Patients: A Practical Workbook. 2009. Available from: http://www.nmhdu.org.uk/silo/files/a-strategy-to-reduce-missing-patients--a-practical-workbook.pdf (accessed 17 April 2014).
- National Patient Safety Agency. *Seven Steps to Patient Safety in Mental Health*. 2008. Available at: http://www.nrls.npsa.nhs.uk/resources/?EntryId45=59858 (accessed 5 November 2013).
- The university of Manchester. National Confidential Inquiry into Suicide and Homicide by People with Mental Illness: Annual Report: England and Wales. July 2009. Available from: http://www.medicine.manchester.ac.uk/psychiatry/research/suicide/prevention/nci/ inquiryannualreports/AnnualReportJuly2009.pdf (accessed 17 April 2014).

Chapter 20: Patient safety in primary care

- Cresswell KM, Panesar SS, Salvilla SA, Carson-Stevens A, Larizgoitia I, Donaldson LJ, Bates D, Sheikh A, World Health Organization's (WHO) Safer Primary Care Expert Working Group. Global research priorities to better understand the burden of iatrogenic harm in primary care: an international delphi exercise. *PLoS Med* 2013;10(11):e1001554.
- Health and Social Care Information Centre. Trends in consultation rates in general practice: 1995–2009. Available at: http://www.hscic.gov.uk/catalogue/PUB01077 (accessed 31 December 2013).
- Sheikh A, Panesar SS, Larizgoitia I, Bates DW, Donaldson LJ. Safer primary care for all: a global imperative. Lancet Glob Health. 2013;1:e182–3
- Zwart DL, Langelaan M, van de Vooren RC, Kuyvenhoven MM, Kalkman CJ, Verheij TJ, Wagner C. Patient safety culture measurement in general practice. Clinimetric properties of 'SCOPE'. *BMC Fam Pract* 2011;12:117.

Chapter 21: Improving the quality of clinical care

- Darzi A. *High Quality Care for All: NHS Next Stage Review.* 2008. Available at: http://webarchive.nationalarchives.gov.uk/+/www.dh.gov.uk/en/Healthcare/Highqualitycareforall/index.htm (accessed 5 November 2013).
- Institute for Healthcare Improvement (IHI). *How to Improve.* 2012. Available at: http://www.ihi.org/knowledge/Pages/Howto-Improve/default.aspx (accessed 5 November 2013).
- Langley G, Moen R, Nolan K, Nolan T, Norman C, Provost L. *The Improvement Guide: A Practical Approach to Enhancing Organizational Performance*, 2nd ed. San Francisco: Jossey-Bass, 2009.

Chapter 22: Science of improvement

- Deming WE. *The New Economics for Industry, Government, and Education*, 2nd ed. Cambridge, MA: MIT Press, 1995.
- Langley G, Moen R, Nolan K, Nolan T, Norman C, Provost L. *The Improvement Guide: A Practical Approach to Enhancing Organizational Performance*, 2nd ed. San Francisco: Jossey-Bass, 2009.
- Maccoby, M, Norman C, Norman J, Margolies R. *Transforming Health Care Leadership*. San Francisco: Jossey-Bass, 2013.

- Perla RJ, Provost LP, Parry GJ. Seven propositions of the science of improvement: exploring foundations. *Qual Manag Health Care* 2013 Jul–Sep; 22(3):170–86.

Chapter 23: Model for Improvement
- Langley G, Moen R, Nolan K, Nolan T, Norman C, Provost L. *The Improvement Guide: A Practical Approach to Enhancing Organizational Performance*, 2nd ed. San Francisco: Jossey-Bass, 2009.

Chapter 24: Measurement for improvement
- Langley G, Moen R, Nolan K, Nolan T, Norman C, Provost L. *The Improvement Guide: A Practical Approach to Enhancing Organizational Performance*, 2nd ed. San Francisco: Jossey-Bass, 2009.
- Perla RJ, Provost LP, Murray SK. Sampling considerations in health care improvement. *Qual Manag Health Care* 2013 Jan–Mar;22(1):36–47.
- Provost LP, Murray SK. *The Health Care Data Guide*. San Francisco, CA: Jossey-Bass, 2011, 264.
- Wheeler DJ, *Understanding variation: the key to managing chaos*, 2nd ed. Knoxville, TN: SPC Press, 2000.

Chapter 25: Spread and sustainability of improvement
- Bosk CL, Dixon-Woods M, Goeschel CA, Pronovost PJ. Reality check for checklists. *Lancet* 2009;374(9688):444–5.
- Dixon-Woods M, Bosk CL, Aveling EL, Goeschel CA, Pronovost PJ. Explaining Michigan: developing an ex post theory of a quality improvement programme. *Milbank Quar* 2011;89(2):167–205.
- Healthcare Improvement Scotland. *Guide on Spread and Sustainability*. 2013. Available at: http://www.healthcareimprovementscotland.org/about_us/what_we_do/knowledge_management/knowledge_management_resources/spread_and_sustainability.aspx (accessed 5 November 2013).
- Health Foundation. Lining up: how do improvement programmes work? Available at: http://www.health.org.uk/publications/lining-up-how-do-improvement-programmes-work/ (accessed 5 November 2013).
- Parry GJ, Carson-Stevens A, Luff DF, McPherson ME, Goldmann DA. Recommendations for the evaluation of health care improvement initiatives. *Acad Pediat* 2013 Nov;13(6):S23–30.

Chapters 26 and 27: Quality improvement tools: visualisation and Quality improvement: assessing the system
- Apkon M, Leonard J, Probst L, *et al*. Design of a safer approach to intravenous drug infusions: failure mode effects analysis. *Qual Saf Health Care* 2004;13(4):265–71.
- Bonfant G, Belfanti P, Paternoster, G, *et al*. Clinical risk analysis with failure mode and effect analysis (FMEA) model in a dialysis unit. *J Nephrol* 2010;23(1):111–18.
- Chiozza ML, Ponzetti, C. FMEA: a model for reducing medical errors. *Clin Chim Acta* 2009; 404(1):75–8.
- Day S, Dalto J, Fox J, Turpin, M. Failure mode and effects analysis as a performance improvement tool in trauma. *J Trauma Nurs* 2006;13(3):111–7.
- de Bucort M, Busse R, Güttler F, *et al*. Process mapping of PTA and stent placement in a university hospital interventional radiology department. *Insights Imaging* 2012;3(4):329–36.
- George ML, Rowlands D, Price M, Maxey J. *The Lean Six Sigma Pocket Toolbook: A Quick Reference Guide to Nearly 100 Tools for Improving Process Quality, Speed, and Complexity*. New York: McGraw-Hill. 2005, 34–48, 145–7, 270–6.
- Johnson JK, Farnan JM, Barach P, *et al*. Searching for the missing pieces between the hospital and primary care: mapping the patient process during care transitions. *BMJ Qual Saf* 2012;21 Suppl 1: i97–105.
- Lago P, Bizzarri G, Scalzotto, F, *et al*. Use of FMEA analysis to reduce risk of errors in prescribing and administering drugs in paediatric wards: a quality improvement project. *BMJ Open* 2012;2(6)1–9.
- Steinberger DM, Douglas SV, Kirschbaum MS. Use of failure mode and effects analysis for proactive identification of communication and handoff failures from organ procurement to transplantation. *Prog Transplant* 2009;19(3):208–14.
- Summers DCS. *Six Sigma Basic Tools and Techniques*. Upper Saddle River, NJ: Pearson, 2007, 105–11, 309–20.
- Trusko BE, Pexton C, Harrington HJ, Gupta PK. *Improving Healthcare Quality and Cost with Six Sigma*. Upper Saddle River, NJ: FT Press, 2007, 118–20.
- van Tilburg CM, Leistikow IP, Rademaker CMA, *et al*. Health care failure mode and effect analysis: a useful proactive risk analysis in a pediatric oncology ward. *Qual Saf Health Care* 2006;15(1):58–64.

Chapter 28: Patient stories in improvement
- 1000Lives+ Stories for Improvement General Resources. http://www.1000livesplus.wales.nhs.uk/stories
- Health Foundation. *Measuring Patient Experience*. 2013. Available at: http://www.health.org.uk/publications/measuring-patient-experience/ (accessed 5 November 2013).
- Patient experiences captured on film. http://healthtalkonline.org
- Patient stories from the Mayo Clinic. http://www.mayoclinic.org/patient-stories
- Patient Stories. Why sorry doesn't have to be the hardest word. 2013. Available at: http://www.patientstories.org.uk/author/murray/page/2/ (accessed 5 November 2013).
- Patient Safety First Leadership for Safety "How to Guide". Using patient stories with Boards. http://www.patientsafetyfirst.nhs.uk/ashx/Asset.ashx?path=/Intervention-support/Patient%20stories%20how%20to%20guide%2020100223.pdf (accessed 5 November 2013).
- Patient voices digital stories. http://www.patientvoices.org.uk/stories.htm

Chapter 29: Leading change in healthcare
- Ajmani K. *Spirit* of a student. 2003. Available at: http://spiritchat.tumblr.com/post/57880016772/students (accessed 5 November 2013).
- Battilana J, Casciaro T. The network secrets of great of change agents. *Harvard Business Review* 2013;91(7). Available at: http://hbr.org/2013/07/the-network-secrets-of-great-change-agents/ar/1 (accessed 15 February 2014).
- Bell C. Fear of learning. 2013. Available at: http://seapointcenter.com/fear-of-learning/ (accessed 5 November 2013).
- Bevan H, Roland D, Lynton J, Jones P, McCrea J. Biggest ever day of collective action to improve healthcare that started with a tweet. Entry, *Hard Business Review*/McKinsey Challenge. 2013. Available at: http://www.mixprize.org/story/biggest-ever-day-collective-action-improve-healthcare-started-tweet-0(accessed 5 November 2013).
- Braithwaite Innovation Group. The thriving individual. 2013. Available at: http://braithwaiteinnovationgroup.com/leadbig/the-thriving-individual/ (accessed 5 November 2013).
- Kelly L. *Rebel, Rebel*. 2013. Available at: http://www.foghound.com/rebel-rebel/ (accessed 5 November 2013).

- Meyerson D. *Tempered Radicals: How Everyday Leaders Inspire Change at Work* Boston, MA: Harvard Business Press, 2003.
- Moore R. Competency model for building and working with system energy. 2011.
- Naseer T. The impact of leaders on personal transformation. 2013. Available at: http://www.tanveernaseer.com/leadership-and-personal-transformation-bill-treasurer/ (accessed 5 November 2013).
- National Advisory Group on the Safety of Patients in England. *A Promise to Learn – a Commitment to Act: Improving the Safety of Patients in England.* London: National Advisory Group, 2013.
- Whyte D. *The Heart Aroused.* New York: Doubleday, 1994.

Chapter 30: Public narrative: story of self, us and now

- Carson-Stevens A, Patel E, Nutt SL, Bhatt J, Panesar SS. The social movement drive: a role for junior doctors in healthcare reform. *J R Soc Med* 2013;106(8):305–9.
- Ganz M. We can be actors, not just spectators. *New Statesman*, 2012. Available at: http://www.newstatesman.com/politics/politics/2012/07/we-can-be-actors-not-just-spectators (accessed 5 November 2013).
- Ganz M. *Why David Sometimes Wins: Leadership, Organization, and Strategy in the California Farm Worker Movement.* New York: Oxford University Press, 2009.

Chapter 31: Planning an improvement project

- Langley G, Moen R, Nolan K, Nolan T, Norman C, Provost L. *The Improvement Guide: A Practical Approach to Enhancing Organizational Performance*, 2nd ed. San Francisco: Jossey-Bass, 2009.
- Institute for Healthcare Improvement (IHI). Open School. Available at: http://www.ihi.org/offerings/IHIOpenSchool/Courses/Pages/Practicum.aspx (accessed 4 January 2014).
- NHS Institute for Innovation and Improvement. Quality and service improvement tools. Available at: http://www.institute.nhs.uk/option,com_quality_and_service_improvement_tools/Itemid,5015.html (accessed 5 November 2013).

Chapter 32: Managing an improvement project

- Agency for Healthcare Research and Quality. Plan-do-study-act (PDSA) cycle. Available at: http://www.innovations.ahrq.gov/content.aspx?id=2398 (accessed 5 November 2013).
- Batalden PB, Davidoff F. Teaching quality improvement: the devil is in the details. *JAMA* 2007;298(9):1059–61.
- Batalden PB, Davidoff F. What is 'quality improvement' and how can it transform healthcare? *Qual Safety Health Care* 2007;16(1):2–3.
- Clark W. *The Gantt Chart: A Working Tool of Management.* New York: Ronald Press Company, 1922.
- Fisher ES, Wennberg DE, Stukel TA, Gottlieb DJ, Lucas FL, Pinder EL. The implications of regional variations in Medicare spending. Part 1: the content, quality, and accessibility of care. *Annals Int Med* 2003;138(4):273–87.
- Fisher ES, Wennberg DE, Stukel TA, Gottlieb DJ, Lucas FL, Pinder EL.The implications of regional variations in Medicare spending. Part 2: health outcomes and satisfaction with care. *Annals Int Med* 2003;138(4):288–98.
- Gardner JW. The nature of leadership. *Leadership Papers* 1987;1.
- Heldman K. *Project Management JumpStart.* 3rd ed. Indianapolis, IN: Sybex, 2011.

- Institute for Healthcare Improvement (IHI). Cause and effect diagram. Available at: http://www.ihi.org/knowledge/Pages/Tools/CauseandEffectDiagram.aspx (accessed 5 November 2013).
- Institute of Medicine (IOM). *Roundtable on Evidence-Based Medicine.* Washington, DC: IOM, 2010.
- James B, Bayley K. *Cost of Poor Quality or Waste in Integrated Delivery System Settings.* Rockville, MD: Agency for Healthcare Research and Quality, 2006.
- Maxwell J. *Developing the Leader within You.* Nashville, TN: Thomas Nelson, 2006.
- NHS Institute for Innovation and Improvement. Quality and service improvement tools. Available at: http://www.institute.nhs.uk/option,com_quality_and_service_improvement_tools/Itemid,5015.html (accessed 5 November 2013).
- Ogrinc GS, Headrick LA. The necessity of process literacy. In: *Fundamentals of Health Care Improvement: A Guide to Improving Your Patients' Care.* Oakbrook Terrace, IL: Joint Commission Resources, 2008, 57–61.
- Pande P, Holpp L. *What Is Six Sigma?* New York, NY: McGraw-Hill, 2002.
- Project Management Institute. Available at: http://www.pmi.org (accessed 5 November 2013).

Chapter 33: Quality improvement in psychiatry

- Bush K, Kivlahan DR, McDonell MB, Fihn SD, Bradley KA. The AUDIT alcohol consumption questions (AUDIT-C): an effective brief screening test for problem drinking. Ambulatory Care Quality Improvement Project (ACQUIP). Alcohol Use Disorders Identification Test. *Arch Intern Med* 1998;158(16):1789–95.
- Frank D, DeBenedetti A, Volk RJ, Williams EC, Kivlahan DR, Bradley KA. Effectiveness of the AUDIT-C as a screening test for alcohol misuse in three race/ethnic groups. *J Gen Intern Med* 2008;23(6):781–7.
- Rosen CS, Kuhn E, Greenbaum MA, Drescher KD. Substance abuse-related mortality among middle-aged male VA psychiatric patients. *Psychiatric Serv* 2008;59(3):290–6.
- World Health Organization. *Global Burden of Mental Disorders and the Need for a Comprehensive, Coordinated Response from Health and Social Sectors at the Country Level.* 2011. Available at: http://apps.who.int/gb/ebwha/pdf_files/EB130/B130_9-en.pdf (accessed 5 November 2013).
- World Health Organization. Global status report on noncommunicable diseases. 2010. Available at: http://www.who.int/nmh/publications/ncd_report_full_en.pdf (accessed 5 November 2013).

Chapter 34: Quality improvement in intensive care

- Department of Health, National Audit Office. *A Safer Place for Patients: Learning to Improve Patient Safety.* HC 456 Session 2005–2006. London: Department of Health, National Audit Office, 2006. Available at: www.nao.org.uk (accessed 5 November 2013).
- Langley G, Moen R, Nolan K, Nolan T, Norman C, Provost L. *The Improvement Guide: A Practical Approach to Enhancing Organizational Performance*, 2nd ed. San Francisco: Jossey-Bass, 2009.

Chapter 35: Quality improvement in obstetrics

- International Federation of Gynecology and Obstetrics. Methodology and tools for quality improvement in maternal and newborn health care. 2011. Available at: http://www.figo.org/journal/methodology-and-tools-quality-improvement-maternal-and-newborn-health-care (accessed 5 November 2013).

Chapter 36: Quality improvement in surgery

• Savory P, Olson J. Guidelines for using process mapping to aid improvement efforts. *Hospital Material Management Quarterly* 2001;22(3):10–6.

Chapter 37: Population health and improvement

• American Public Health Association. Quality improvement initiatives. Available at: http://www.apha.org/programmes/standards/ (accessed 5 November 2013).

• Institute for Healthcare Improvement (IHI). Triple aim initiative. Available at: http://www.ihi.org/offerings/Initiatives/TripleAIM/Pages/default.aspx (accessed 31 December 2013).

• Jain N, Keeney R. Strategic quality improvement imperative: population health management. In *Patient Safety and Quality Healthcare 2013*. Available at: http://www.psqh.com/online-first/1577-strategic-quality-improvement-imperative-population-health-management.html (accessed 5 November 2013).

• Pracilio VP, Reifsnyder J, Nash DB, Fabius RJ. The population health mandate. In: Nash D, Reifsnyder J, Fabius R, Pracilio V, eds. Population health: Creating a culture of wellness. Sudbury, Massachusetts: Jones and Bartlett; 2011:xxxv-lii.

• Stiefel M, Nolan K. *A Guide to Measuring the Triple Aim: Population Health, Experience of Care, and Per Capita Cost*. IHI Innovation Series white paper. Cambridge, MA: Institute for Healthcare Improvement; 2012. Available at: http://www.ihi.org/knowledge/Pages/IHIWhitePapers/AGuidetoMeasuringTripleAim.aspx (accessed 5 November 2013).

Index

Patient Safety and Healthcare Improvement at a Glance, First Edition. Edited by Sukhmeet S. Panesar, Andrew Carson-Stevens, Sarah A. Salvilla and Aziz Sheikh
© 2014 John Wiley & Sons, Ltd. Published 2014 by John Wiley & Sons, Ltd.